HEAL YOUR
HUNGER

HEAL YOUR
HUNGER

7 Simple Steps to **End Emotional Eating** Now

Tricia Nelson

Host of the *Heal Your Hunger Show*

HEAL YOUR HUNGER
7 Simple Steps to End Emotional Eating Now

First Printing: 2017
Printed in USA

Graphic Design by Adele Wiejaczka

HEAL YOUR HUNGER, INC.
11740 San Vicente Blvd. Suite 109-200
Los Angeles, CA 90049
800.609.4061

www.HealYourHunger.com

ORDERING INFORMATION
Special discounts are available on quantity purchases by corporations, associations, educators, and others. For details, contact the publisher at the above listed address.

BOOKING, PRESS & SPEAKING INQUIRIES
www.HealYourHunger.com/Contact

DEDICATION

To my best friend and greatest inspiration, Roy Nelson.

how to
READ THIS
book

You will find some of this book's most important concepts in large type so you can flip through and grab some juicy morsels right away. Enjoy!

You'll also find a host of "goodies"—cheat sheets, worksheets, and a special training video—that summarize and serve as a companion to the chapters. It will also make reading this book even easier.

You can access this bonus information right now at
www.healyourhungerbook.com.

Beyond that, while you may be tempted to skip ahead and read the chapters that speak to you most, I hope you'll start at the beginning and read through to the end.

There is an intentional flow to this book, with each chapter building on the last, to form a foundation of understanding that will support you and actually begin to heal you as you read.

Allow that flow to happen by reading the chapters in order. As you read, you will experience a transformation in your perspective—and in your relationship with food.

I am super excited for this to happen for you!

Use all the tools offered in this book and in the bonus materials, and you'll find that your path to heal your hunger is well under way.

If you want help to implement what's in this book, I've created a companion course, **10 Weeks to Freedom from Emotional Eating**. You can learn more about this through the bonus link above.

table of
CONTENTS

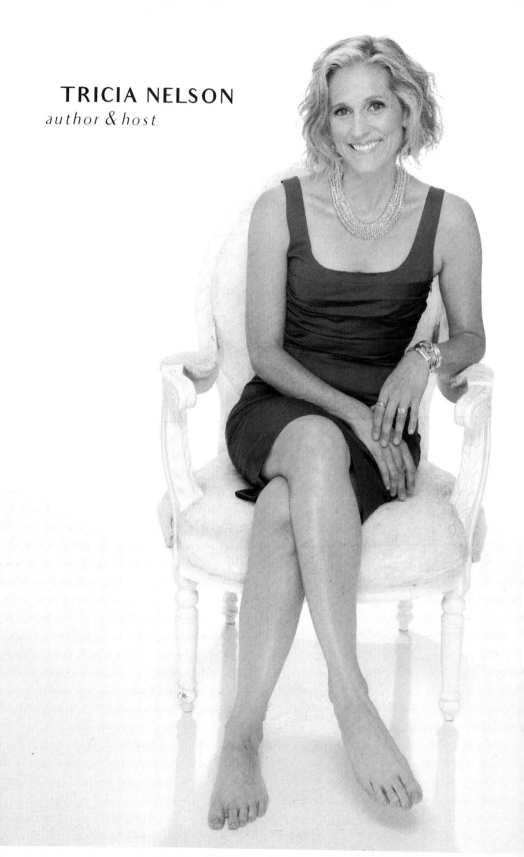

TRICIA NELSON
author & host

why i
WROTE
this book

I WROTE THIS BOOK FOR YOU.

If you're one of the millions of people struggling with food and weight, I know exactly how you feel. I've been there, so I understand firsthand how painful, frustrating, and demoralizing it can be. And like you, I've learned, mostly the hard way, that when it comes to ending the battle with weight, most of the solutions out there just don't work.

More to the point, they don't work for people like *us*.

I wrote *Heal Your Hunger* so I could speak to the person closest to my heart: the emotional eater. YOU. Of course, you might not be sure that the term "emotional eater" applies to you. There was a time when I didn't relate to the term at all. I wasn't an emotional eater—I just liked food! I liked to think about it, cook it, eat it, serve it to others. Anything having to do with food, you could count me in.

So if you have troubles with food or weight but aren't sure about the "emotional" part, I hope you'll stay with me here. I want to help shed some light on this generally misunderstood topic.

Sure, we've all met someone who went on a diet, dropped ten or twenty pounds, and never looked back. Or that one in a million who struggled with their weight, picked up an activity such as, say, marathon running, fell in love with it, and completely changed their body and their life.

But those success stories—the verifiable ones, anyway—are exceedingly rare. How do I know? Well, here are a few statistics worth pondering:

- Close to 70 percent of American adults are either overweight or obese. (That's seven out of ten people.)
- Each year, about 45 million people in this country go on a diet.
- US consumers spend $109 million *every day* on diet and weight-loss products.
- Annually, weight loss is a $60 billion industry.
- Right now, on Amazon, there are 65,000 weight-loss books and 365,000 fitness books.

And yet, 98 percent of all diets fail. That means that out of every hundred people who go on a diet, only two will lose weight and keep it off. Of course, you probably already know something about that.

Look back over your life and think about how many diets you've tried. How many times have you tried to control your eating? How long have you stood on the scales, trying to will them into giving you a lower number?

How many diets has it been? Was it the grapefruit diet, the Scarsdale diet, the Atkins diet, the Beverly Hills diet, the South Beach diet, the Jillian Michaels diet, the cookie diet, the low-carb, no-carb, or all-the-carbs-you-want diet?

How many exercise programs, gyms, and aerobics classes have you tried?

Now, pause for a moment and ask yourself this:

How many more diets and exercise programs do I have to go on before I realize that they are not the solution to my food and weight issue?

And more importantly, if they aren't the solution, *what is?*

That is what this book is all about.

You may have given up even trying to find a solution. You may have decided it's just too hard. You can't bear being disappointed one more time. You've seen it all, and now you are jaded and despondent. You've decided it's not worth trying to be thin—too much heartache, too much shame when you fail. Too much self-loathing after one more time that you've spent a bunch of money, dared to hope, and then ended up in the same place you always do: bingeing and fat. Again.

I want you to know that there really is hope. You can get past your issues with food and weight *once and for all*. I know because I've done it, and I have no more willpower than you. And I've been privileged to see hundreds of other people do it, too.

In fact, you will be comforted by reading this book even if you're not overweight but still have issues with food or weight. This book is for you if you ever grapple with . . .

- binge eating
- restricting
- purging
- regurgitation
- constant dieting
- food obsession, or
- exercise fanaticism.

ANYTHING THAT MUST BE CONTROLLED IS ALREADY OUT OF CONTROL.

These problems may all seem different to you, but they all involve an obsession with food and weight. They all reflect various phases of control (or lack of it). And usually, anything that must be controlled is already out of control. So the compulsion to overeat is what drives all these people, no matter what their body size or eating patterns. Wherever you fall on the disordered-eating spectrum—whether you're a restrictor rationing bites of a single Larabar, or a binge eater consuming volumes of food in one evening—you are manifesting a *symptom* of one overriding issue: *emotional eating*. And solving it is about much more than changing what you eat, the way you eat, or how much you weigh.

If you're not sure whether you are an emotional eater, or if you think you are, but aren't sure your problem actually qualifies as "food addiction," I've created a little quiz that will help you know for sure. You will receive a personalized score that indicates where you are on the emotional eating/food addiction spectrum.

You can find this quiz at www.healyourhungerbook.com.

If you are an emotional eater, no matter where you land on the spectrum, this book will benefit you. I was fifty pounds overweight and was both an emotional eater and a food addict. I never had an "off" button once I took that first compulsive bite—that bite that I didn't need but wanted simply because I was compelled. And once I started to eat in a compulsive way, it was over. I was rolling downhill with no brakes. I couldn't close the bag or put the lid on the carton. One piece of candy or one cookie was never enough for me. If more was available, I ate it. This is what made me different from "normal eaters": the inability to stop myself.

Everything you will read in these pages comes from my personal struggles with—and eventual healing from—problems with food and weight. I also have close to thirty years of experience helping others overcome their battle with emotional eating and food addiction. So you're in the right place. I'm not here to talk down to you or lecture you, *because we are the same, you and I.* I've been where you are, and I'm here to offer real hope and a simple, effective solution.

WHAT IS EMOTIONAL EATING?

If this is a new concept to you, you may be wondering what, exactly, emotional eating is. Simple: *It is using food to quiet (stuff) emotions.*

Put another way, emotional eating is using food to meet needs beyond physical nourishment. What kinds of needs?

1. SOCIAL NEEDS

Emotional eaters use food to feel better when they're lonely—for example, if we're alone after a breakup, or at home feeling bored on a Saturday night. We also use it when we're anxious and uncomfortable around other people—say, at a party or social event. We use food to give us a boost of confidence when we're feeling insecure, in the same way that an alcoholic uses "liquid courage." For many of us, food made us feel more jovial and outgoing—right up until it backfired and made us feel isolated and separate. Food was the social lubricant that made getting along in this world seem easier. (Again, until it ultimately made everything much, much harder!)

2. EMOTIONAL NEEDS

Emotional eaters use food for comfort and companionship. Dealing with people isn't easy for us, so we resort to the ease of getting emotional support from something that never seems to let us down, never rejects us, and is always available: food. Food is not only a loyal friend, but a protector as well. For those of us who have been sexually abused, food seems to protect us from the attention and unwanted advances of others. We literally build walls of fat to keep people away for years, sometimes decades. Ultimately, though, those walls turn out to be a prison instead of a fortress, keeping us trapped in a private hell that we fear we may never escape.

3. MENTAL NEEDS

Emotional eaters often suffer from an "overactive" or "racing" mind. We use food to distract ourselves from all the thoughts and worries that keep us worked up and on edge. Our mind dashes at warp speed in all directions, and we can't slow down no matter how many things we try. Settling down with a pint of Ben & Jerry's and a box of shortbread cookies often does the trick—at least, for a few hours. When we're drunk on food, we can forget the cares of the day. We numb out and aren't bothered by anything.

4. SPIRITUAL NEEDS

It may surprise you how many emotional eaters are spiritual seekers. We have spent years exploring spirituality and trying to make a connection that can bring us comfort, lessen our fear, and help us control our eating. We have a deep craving for meaning, for an understanding of our greater pur-pose, and for a feeling of oneness and well-being. And because we don't know how to achieve this, we resort to food—at first as an attempt to satisfy that yearning, and eventually to forget that we ever felt that yearning to begin with.

Of course, emotional eaters come in all shapes and sizes; but we have this in common: we use the obsession with food to treat our emotions. Whether you're heavy or thin, male or female, gay or straight, you use food, in some way, to stuff your emotions.

I wrote this book to help stir your consciousness, to rouse you out of the deep slumber of denial and neglect that has overtaken you during years of habitual eating and avoiding your emotional self. I want to help you awaken to the truth about why you overeat, and show you how to finally stop. I want to help you understand what's really going on when you feel hungry. And then I want to help you identify and adopt new ways of feeding yourself—physically, emotionally, and spiritually. I want to show you how to heal your hunger for good, so that you never again have to live as a slave to food.

I must warn you up front that this book may not be an easy one to read. It may stir up emotions in you that you didn't expect. To get at the real source of your hunger, I'll be pushing you to dig a little deeper than you may be used to going, and this could get uncomfortable. After all, I'm here to challenge your beliefs and ideas about weight loss, food, and yourself. Our goal here is to demystify the entire concept of emotional eating, so that you have new clarity, new insight, and new tools that will empower you to take decisive, effective action. We can use my experience—both the painful, torturous experience of living as an out-of-control eater, and my path of healing and helping others heal—as a catalyst for change and a beacon of light to illuminate your own path of healing.

You've taken a huge first step by picking up this book and reading this far into it. Kudos to you! I suggest you use this book as a reference guide, not just as something to read once and be done with. You'll get the most out of it if you keep it close by and reread it from time to time. Also, because this is such a behemoth of a topic, I chose what I consider the most important advice about how to end emotional eating, but there's much more to share with you. (After all, I wanted the book to be short enough that you'd read it!) So I've put together a training, useful links, and several cheat sheets and that will help guide you as you read this book. I encourage you to access this bonus information as it will help you assimilate what's in this book, as well as give you an opportunity to go deeper.

You can access your bonus materials now at www.healyourhungerbook.com.

Okay, ready to get started? Then let's go!

PART 1

THE CRAZY REALITY
of the
EMOTIONAL EATER

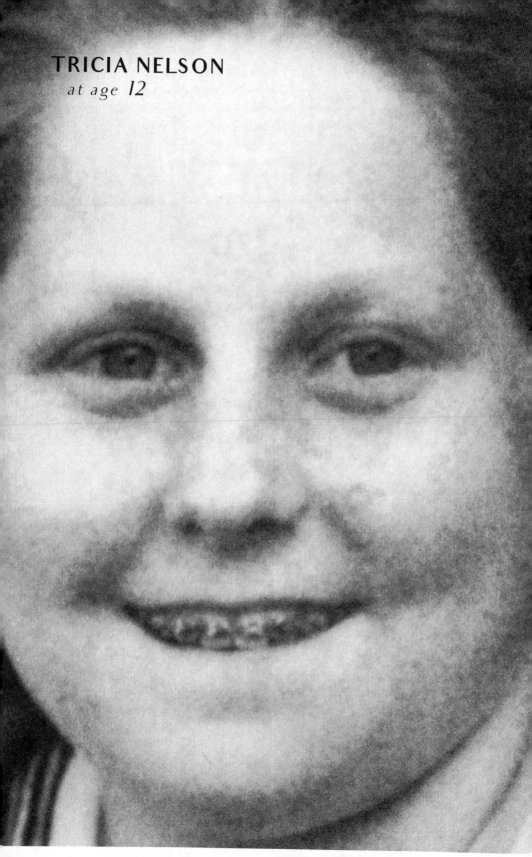

TRICIA NELSON
at age 12

my STORY

I grew up as a fat girl, which was very painful. I hated my body. My tummy was one big roll of fat that I would scrunch up and hold in my hands—with disgust. I imagined slicing it off in the same way that my dad would slice the fat off the edge of a steak! I would also fantasize about getting some kind of disease that would make me lose weight without trying, or joining the army so I'd be forced to exercise at Boot Camp. (I hated exercise, so this was the only way I could imagine myself doing it.)

I also had a lot of fear. I was terribly afraid, even though I didn't really have anything to fear from the world around me. I grew up in a good home in Concord, Massachusetts. My parents were happily married and provided well for us, and we traveled and spent summers in Maine. It was all good—on the outside.

But inside, where I lived, I was hurting.

Of course, I wasn't always aware on a conscious level that I was hurting. I was a happy-go-lucky kid who laughed a lot, had friends, and was active in theater and music. I had a paper route to make money and pursued creative projects. My friend Molly and I were quite the budding entrepreneurs with our barrette-painting business in seventh and eighth grade. It was great fun.

But under that happy facade, I was burying pain and shame that I couldn't talk about with *anyone*. Like the sexual abuse from a relative when I was young. That was a dark secret I kept entirely to myself. Then there was the embarrassment over being so fat that my legs chafed when I ran, being afraid of the dark, and masturbating compulsively whenever I was alone in the house.

I couldn't open up to anyone about any of this.

When I was fifteen, my oldest sister told me she ate because of her emotions. I thought that was the craziest thing I'd ever heard! *I just liked food.* Yet the seed was planted, and over the next few years, I began to notice that my relationship with food wasn't normal. Food was far more important to me than it was to others.

BUT UNDER THAT HAPPY FACADE, I WAS BURYING PAIN AND SHAME.

For instance, whenever my friends and I went to Friendly's restaurant after school, some of my friends would invariably leave french fries on their plate after eating their burger. I couldn't imagine doing that. After all, the french fries were the best part!

Some would eat half a hot fudge sundae and just stop, saying, "I'm full!" I would think, *What does "full" have to do with anything?*

Despite my preoccupation with food, I did okay. I was elected president of my high school; I played varsity sports; I got good enough grades—I did everything I was supposed to do. I was accepted to one of the top colleges in the country. Everything seemed good on the outside . . . except for my weight.

On the inside, things weren't so great. I couldn't quiet the fear. I would eat to cope with my feelings, stuffing myself with food, often to the point where I felt sick. Sometimes, I would even fish food out of the garbage after throwing it away. I would binge to the point of disgust, toss out the food I couldn't finish, and pass out in front of the T.V. Then a few hours later, when I wasn't quite as full, I'd renegotiate my decision and go get the food I had thrown out!

I went on diets, joined a gym, tried to starve myself (I could last only half a day), and forced myself to jog—which I hated doing more than anything in the world.

By the time I was eighteen, I knew that no matter how hard I tried, I couldn't change my eating patterns or my weight on my own. I finally gave up on diets and exercise after I spent an entire summer dieting and jogging every day and only managed, at a height of five feet six, to fluctuate between 150 and 155 pounds. Looking back, I think it was the snacking!

After high school, I sought help from a twelve-step program that dealt with food issues, and I also started therapy. *But neither of these things helped me change my eating.* I still battled food and my weight constantly.

After two years in college, I decided to take time off from school and move to the other side of the country. I realize now that I was just trying to get away from myself and my family. I had a lot of unresolved issues with my family—mostly resentment and anger—and I thought that by moving away geographically, I could leave it all behind. Well, anyone who has tried knows that it doesn't quite work that way.

By the time I moved, I had reached 170 pounds. I continued with the twelve-step program, and this time I sought help from an eating-disorder therapist, whom I saw twice a week. By now, I had a whole shelf of self-help books and workbooks. I always held out hope that just around the corner there was something that would work for me. And yet, nothing I tried was doing it for me—and I tried everything. Of course, I learned a lot, but all the knowledge in the world couldn't stop me from bingeing. The compulsion and obsession with food just wouldn't stop.

I THOUGHT THAT BY MOVING AWAY GEOGRAPHICALLY, I COULD LEAVE IT ALL BEHIND.

And my deep-seated sense of worthlessness continued to haunt me. It wreaked havoc in my life every day, in the form of self-sabotaging choices around men, money, and friendships. My friendships were usually very one-sided, with me putting in all the effort and getting little in return. No matter how hard I tried to create a life for myself, I could never make it happen.

I had no idea what to do about it. After all, I was doing what seemed like all the right things, but they just weren't working for me.

At the age of twenty-one, I was really starting to despair. After I lost a bunch of weight using a strict eating plan, the weight loss went straight to my head. I became obsessed with my body and couldn't get enough hits from feeling and looking thin. I loved it when people noticed and made comments. I finally fit into normal-size clothes, so I would change outfits three times in a day! Without the food to fill me, I would stuff myself with other distractions: self-obsession, shopping for clothes, and *men*.

I was constantly in and out of relationships. Since I was afraid of intimacy, I preferred the "chase" and the initial "honeymoon/obsession" stage of a relationship to actually *being in a relationship*. I also always went too fast sexually because I couldn't say no. So as soon as things got intimate (which was always too soon), I would find something wrong with the guy and be off and running again, looking for my next victim.

The end result of all this chaos is that I eventually felt so uncomfortable in my own skin that I started craving my old friend, food. In no time at all, I was off to the races, and the number on the scales started creeping upward.

I thought, *I can't keep this up, yo-yoing up and down twenty to fifty pounds for the rest of my life.* There had to be a better way.

But I was doing everything I knew how to do. What was I missing?

Finally, two women I knew from our mutual battles with food and weight seemed to find the answer. One had been hopelessly bulimic and couldn't stop bingeing and purging for a single day. She had been obese, lost the weight, and became bulimic as she fought to control the effects of her recurring binges. No one could help her, and she had looked everywhere.

One day, I saw her, and she seemed different. She explained that her obsession and compulsion were lifted and she wasn't bulimic anymore. She said that a few weeks earlier, *she had lost the desire to binge and purge.* The difference was amazing. Indeed, I almost didn't recognize her—that's how dramatic the change was. I had to wonder, what was her secret?

A few days later, I ran into another woman who had the same kind of experience. And she told me the most astounding thing. *Both she and the bulimic woman were receiving help from the same person.* They were working with a man who was doing what no one else could: helping them eliminate not just extra pounds, not just their issues with weight, but their entire obsession with food.

I said, "Give me his number. I have to talk to this guy *now.*"

I raced home and called Roy Nelson. I scheduled a time to meet with him and actually drove to another city that very day to visit with him. And though it may sound dramatic, my life has never been the same since.

Roy taught me about this terrible condition that is food addiction. He showed me, clearly and indelibly, that all my efforts to lose weight, when they came from the outside (diets, gyms, pills and potions, even therapy and twelve-step programs focused on food and weight loss), were never going to save me.

Roy told me that food was not my problem, and neither was weight. These were just symptoms of my problem. And I had to admit that deep in my heart, I knew this, because I had proved it over and over again through my many failures.

This book is my way of sharing with you what Roy taught me about the true causes of my emotional eating and food addiction. I want you to learn from my path of healing. I'm excited to share the research and experiences I've gathered through the extraordinary privilege of working alongside Roy for close to thirty years to help people heal their addiction to food. I have witnessed miracles in hundreds of people's lives—people who once felt just like me.

And maybe even just like you.

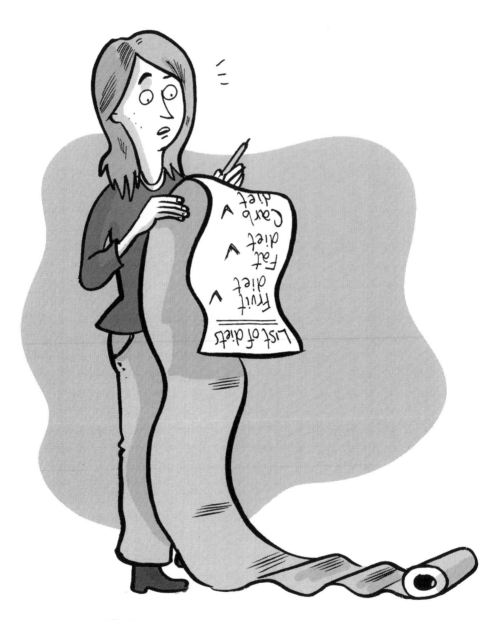

EVERYTHING WE'VE TRIED...

© 2017 by Tricia Nelson

why NOTHING *you've tried has* WORKED

If picking up this book is the very first thing you've ever done in the hope of dealing with your food issues, congratulations. You just saved yourself a lot of time and disappointment. You have taken the first step in overcoming your problem, without sinking years, money, and hope in things that, ultimately, just don't work.

If, on the other hand, you're like most people reading this book right now (and like me), you know firsthand what a demoralizing and exhausting path trying to control out-of-control eating can be. You've probably tried several methods that, at least initially, seemed as though they would help you take charge of your eating once and for all. You've probably tried diet and exercise. Maybe you've invested in diet pills, potions, and lotions. Perhaps you've read books, attended twelve-step programs, dabbled in therapy, experimented with hypnosis—maybe even resorted to surgery.

And don't get me wrong: some of these things have done wonders—for *some* people.

But why haven't they worked for you? It's not because you're fundamentally flawed and ultimately to blame for your problems. The fact that you can't "get it" doesn't mean there's something wrong with you.

The methods you've tried over the span of your lifetime haven't worked, for the simple reason that they *couldn't* work. They weren't designed to deal with the problem you're suffering from, which has nothing to do with food.

I'm sorry to say, you've been barking up the wrong tree. But there is an approach that might answer the question "Why can't I get it?" and that can finally help you live the kind of life that, at this point, you probably don't dare imagine. Before exploring that life, though, let's take a closer look at why the things you've tried haven't worked.

THE LIST

DIETS AND EXERCISE

For the overwhelming majority, diets and exercise are the first place people turn when they want to lose weight. On the face of it, it makes sense to attack the problem in the quickest, most direct way possible. Of course, when we decide to go on a diet, many of us develop a sort of situational amnesia and forget the twenty diets that have already bombed.

Adding to the problem is the fact that the "diet and exercise" solution is regarded as irrefutable conventional wisdom. This is what the doctors have to offer us. And they're the experts! It makes perfect sense, right? Consume fewer calories and burn more—this is how you lose weight. It's simple arithmetic.

THE FACT THAT YOU CAN'T "GET IT" DOESN'T MEAN THERE'S SOMETHING WRONG WITH YOU.

Unless you happen to be an emotional eater—which most people struggling with weight are, whether they realize it or not.

Not that the advice to eat less and exercise more is wrong—it isn't. Physiologically, that is how one loses weight. But when you're an emotional eater, when you are addicted to food, you *can't* "just eat less." That's like asking an alcoholic to simply "drink less." If you know anything about alcoholics, you know how well that works!

Dieting is a trap for emotional eaters. Sure, it's good to put a cap on food intake and have some structure around meals. But it's never sustainable when imposed from the outside. When emotional eaters go on a diet, they no longer have extra food to lean on when life gets tough. So while they may feel high from losing weight, they also tend to feel on edge and bitchy. They don't have their primary means of coping with stress, so they become miserable. (And those around them may, also.)

When they are miserable long enough, they get fed up and go right back to the ease and comfort of excessive eating.

The bottom line is, diets aren't sustainable. If you go on a diet, you must eventually go off the diet. Weight loss has to be a natural result of needing less food emotionally, combined with an organic desire to treat your body and mind in a healthier way. If it isn't, then it's only a matter of time before you break out and return to your old patterns. The change in eating habits has to come from within.

And the "exercise more" part of the equation isn't any easier. It's hard to feel motivated to exercise when you're stuffed from bingeing, have no motivation, and feel down in the dumps. The last thing a sedentary, obese person wants to do is exercise! That's why the only way they'll do it is if Jillian Michaels (of *The Biggest Loser* fame) is in their face, yelling at them.

THE CHANGE IN EATING HABITS HAS TO COME FROM WITHIN.

I don't mean to suggest that exercise is not a great thing. Our bodies must have exercise to be optimally healthy. Exercise helps prevent negative health conditions and diseases, improves your mood, boosts your energy, enhances your sleep, improves your sex life, and can even be fun (though maybe not at first).

For emotional eaters, the problem with exercise is that we usually do it for the wrong reasons. We may pay lip service to doing it to be healthy, but we do it to lose weight, even when we say we're not. We look at it as a tradeoff, thinking we'll be able to eat more because of the calories we've spent. So while we may exercise to lose weight, we end up exercising so we can eat more.

Then we end up eating far more than we expended in energy, which totally defeats the purpose (our purpose, anyway) for exercising in the first place!

PILLS, POTIONS, AND SUPPLEMENTS

People have been taking diet pills for ages. Why? Because they appeal to our "quick fix" mentality and our fantastical thinking. ("Yes, Virginia, there is a magical way to be able to eat whatever you want and still lose weight.") No wonder diet pills are a $40 billion industry. We've been seduced by the notion that we can indeed have our cake and eat it, too. In fact, we can even have it à la mode.

Emotional eaters are willing to believe anything if it means we can still eat and lose weight. Our dependence on food is so great that we are regularly and willingly suckered by every weight-loss lie out there.

And the pills-and-potions arena is a breeding ground for weight-loss lies. The few supplements that actually do help us stay healthy are one thing, but diet pills, diuretics, "fat-blocking" medications—they're all the same trap in different guises. The mind of an emotional eater is already playing tricks, maneuvering and justifying how they can eat more without consequence. So anything that plays into this myth that we can lose weight without eating less or dealing with the underlying emotional causes is simply a setup for more failure.

Why do diet pills fail? Because as emotional eaters, we always overeat anyway. We need food on an emotional level, so no matter what appetite suppressant we take; we still want our fix. Medications may help a bit, for a time. But since an emotional eater's hunger usually isn't physical, the powders and pills can never sate it.

FOOD IS NOT THE PROBLEM. FOOD IS A SYMPTOM AND WHAT WE USE TO TREAT THE PROBLEM.

So while the high of a new product or gimmick can make you feel (for a while, anyway) as if it were working, that's usually placebo effect, or it's the euphoria of starting something new. Or it's because you finally started doing *something* positive for yourself. We've all started diets and felt excited. We tell ourselves, "This is it! This time I'm really going to do this thing." We've all been through that a hundred or a thousand times. But as long as it's all based on treating the *symptom* of food and weight, it won't stand the test of time.

To be clear: food is not the problem. Food is a symptom and what we use to treat the problem.

TWELVE-STEP PROGRAMS

Twelve-step programs are certainly a big move up from miracle pills and potions. They provide fellowship with people who suffer from the same addiction, which helps us realize that we're not alone in our suffering and experience. The twelve steps are spiritual in nature, and they can have a profound effect on your perspective and can relieve the compulsion to use an addiction. In a perfect world, the twelve-step programs would heal every one of us of whatever problems we have, and there would be no need for any other approach.

And then there's this world—the one we actually live in.

To give you a little history, Overeaters Anonymous is the "grandmother" of all the food-related twelve-step programs. At one time, it was all there was. But because so many people attended OA for years without actually experiencing much weight loss, some got frustrated and decided they needed more focus on food and weight-loss success. So other programs eventually spun off from OA. These include GreySheeters Anonymous, CEA-HOW, Food Addicts Anonymous, Food Addicts in Recovery Anonymous, and so on. The difference between the spin-offs is based primarily on differences of opinion on what "food plan" to follow. GreySheeters has a diet that is different from FA's. CEA-HOW's is different from either, and Food Addicts in Recovery has yet another diet.

There are many people who have experienced life-changing recovery in these programs. Many others, unfortunately, continue to slip and slide. While these programs are intended to address much more than physical weight loss, too often there's a hyper-focus on food and weight, which misses the point. Anytime

ANYTIME I DID PUT DOWN THE FOOD, I JUST ENDED UP SUBSTITUTING OTHER ADDICTIONS.

we focus too much on food, weight, measuring cups and scales, we can easily overlook the real problem: the emotional underpinnings that drive our need to eat. When these go unaddressed, "abstinence" from overeating becomes hard and uncomfortable and, ultimately, impossible. So we overeat. This is why the twelve-step programs become a revolving door for people who tried it, had some success for a time, and then eventually "fell off the wagon"—just like those in the diet-and-exercise camp.

I was someone who just couldn't quite get it. I would abstain from compulsive eating for a time and then, eventually, break out and begin overeating again. So I ended up yo-yoing in Overeaters Anonymous just as much as I had yo-yoed before I went to OA—not the effect I was looking for.

And anytime I did put down the food, I just ended up substituting other addictions. Jonesing for a fix I would turn to more "acceptable" options: diet soda, gum, cigarettes, shopping, sex—you name it, I tried it. I had to have something to quell the nervousness and racing mind. I was so uncomfortable without my food, I had to bury my feelings in other ways.

But those substitute fixes never really did the trick. I would always end up over-eating, and the cycle would begin all over again.

Ultimately, it became clear that I had to heal at a deeper level, that just below the surface of my overeating and weight gain was a lot of pain. And without addressing it, I would be consigning myself to a lifetime of struggle—in or out-side the twelve-step rooms.

THERAPY

If you're beginning to accept the idea that your eating is, in fact, emotional, you may think that seeing a therapist is the logical, effective way to deal with the problem. And there are some wonderfully insightful and talented therapists in the world. Unfortunately, though, if you are addicted to food, the therapeutic model will rarely be enough to stop you from overeating. Therapy is valuable because it can help a person open up about their problems in a confidential setting and, hopefully, identify solutions. The main benefit is the revelation part of the process—you become aware of your actions and feelings during therapy so that you can then make changes in your behavior.

The problem is, when it comes to food addiction, awareness is not enough. Being aware of something on an intellectual level does not produce healing on an emotional level. The fears and patterns behind our behavior don't get better just because we understand them. This is primarily because these deeper issues are lodged within our subconscious minds, and *we can't change our subconscious with intellectual understanding.* Our subconscious doesn't respond to that.

THE SUBCONSCIOUS MIND CAN BE CHANGED ONLY BY MEANS OF THE HEART.

The subconscious mind can be changed only by means of the heart, which is the threshold of the subconscious. Deep within the heart lie our hopes and our aspirations, feelings of deep love as well as all the fear and pain we have buried over our lifetime. The same fear and pain are the foundation of the untrue beliefs that lurk in our subconscious and motivate many of our self-defeating decisions.

I spent years in therapy hoping to heal the buried fears and pain. But because I was approaching it from an intellectual basis, my head was engaged without my heart being sufficiently opened. To move beyond intellectual reasoning about a problem, to an experience of deeper healing of that problem, we must have access to the heart. And in my experience, we can access our hearts only when we feel deep safety and love. The therapeutic model can indeed provide a feeling of safety and sometimes love, but for the addict, part of that safety happens only when there is a connection at the *heart level.* And that connection is possible only when one person who has experienced healing from food addiction is connecting with one who hasn't but wants to. Again, the only thing that can dislodge problems of pain, fear, and guilt in the subconscious is the healing power of love. Our hearts must be open and trusting, and the identification with those who have been "been there" helps foster that trust.

SURGERY

Surgery takes the allure of the "quick fix" to a whole new level. Surgical options such as liposuction, gastric bypass surgery, Lap-Band surgery, and plastic surgery are expensive and invasive and carry a significant element of risk. In some cases, they can even be life threatening.

Never mind that surgery is a desperate way to try to control the effects of emotional eating without getting anywhere near the root of the problem. Many people who have tried these extreme forms of control contact us because, even with their altered bodies, they are *still* plagued by an uncontrollable urge to overeat. You can surgically alter your stomach size, but when was the size of your stomach ever a consideration during a food binge? Singer and TV personality Carnie Wilson is an obvious example of this phenomenon. She regained the weight she lost after gastric bypass surgery, and twelve years later, she went under the knife again in hopes of a better result. She's not the only one to try it more than once.

Such is the sense of desperation and denial that drives this condition.

People who had this surgery and then put some or most of the weight back on have told me they simply got more creative in finding ways to get their fix. From milkshakes to popcorn to alcohol, they did whatever it took to get the emotional relief they needed.

HYPNOSIS

Hypnosis has helped some addicts break habits such as smoking. But for something as complex as emotional eating, hypnosis rarely works, especially over the long term. The underlying issues that drive food addiction are too powerful to be healed through hypnosis. Even if the cravings are temporarily relieved—which they can be—the underlying issues will still be there, leading to other problems, which usually include relapse.

SUBSTITUTION

We touched on this earlier. Some emotional eaters actually view trading their food obsession for something that doesn't affect their weight as a positive solution. Think of people who go on a diet and take up smoking cigarettes to satisfy their oral fixation, or they get fanatical about exercise, becoming compulsive marathon runners, triathletes, or "workoutaholics."

Some experts actually encourage addicts to substitute addictions. Distracting ourselves from temptation and becoming obsessed with a healthy activity is indeed preferable to overeating. But how long can that distraction really last? How long can hot yoga fill the empty place inside that we used to fill with food? Over time, the exercise enthrallment will pale and those dark places will emerge again, nagging for a stronger form of relief.

ACCEPTANCE

Most people who are overweight and try for years to gain control—typically in the ways we've looked at in this chapter—at some point finally give up trying. They are so sick of failing that to protect themselves from further disappointment, they say, "I don't care anymore. I'm just going to accept myself the way that I am." Or "I'm not meant to be thin."

Maybe you're one of them.

If so, you probably don't *want* to accept yourself this way—you'd give anything to be thin—but since you can't get there, you stop trying. So you try to settle into what is often referred to as "fat serenity."

WHAT WE RESIST FORCES US, AND WHAT WE FORCE RESISTS US.

"Fat serenity" is not the same thing as acceptance. Accepting our bodies as they are is essential, because fighting how we are will only keep us stuck there. What we resist forces us, and what we force resists us.

But there is a difference between *accepting* our weight and *settling* for our weight. To change something, we must first accept that it is the way it is. If a coffee table is brown and we pretend it's red, it can't ever *be* red until we first get honest about the fact that it's brown. So coming to terms with our weight is a big step, especially since a major factor of this condition is denial.

There are people who really don't care that they are fat. They have been overweight all their lives, everyone in their family is overweight, and their friends and most people in their town are overweight, so there doesn't seem to be anything wrong with it. If you've ever seen an installment of the TV series *Here Comes Honey Boo Boo*, you know what I'm talking about. There are people who just don't have that angst about their weight. They may care when they start being restricted physically because of their weight, but it's really not a burning issue.

Since you are reading this book, it's probably safe to assume that you do care and that you want to make a change. But it's still essential that you start by accepting your body as it is right now. Accepting that you have a problem is a very different thing from settling for a life with that problem.

In my case, if I had "settled in" to being obese, I would never have experienced the freedom I have today. Luckily, that was never really an option. I was terribly unhappy with my weight and obsessed with finding a way to change it. I had to accept it as my current reality, to be sure, but I couldn't accept it as the way it should be or even the way it was okay to be—because for me, it just wasn't.

If you're like me—if you're someone who is really bothered by your weight, if you feel plagued by worry, embarrassment, and shame about your weight (even if you're not overweight at all)—consider yourself lucky. That pain you feel about your weight is what prompted you to pick up this book even after reading fifty others. That angst keeps you searching and hoping for a solution. That angst has led you here, to a new approach to your problem.

I believe from the depths of my soul that being thin is the natural order of things. If you think about it, it makes perfect sense. We gain weight when we eat more calories than the body can burn. This means, essentially, that we are eating too much. And if we are overeating, if we are eating food that our bodies don't need in order to function, there's a reason.

That reason is usually emotional. So it makes sense that if we stop the emotional eating—provided there is not a medical issue, such as a reaction to medication, that is keeping the weight on (which is fairly rare)—we will lose weight. Even without exercising. (Heresy, I know!)

PRAYER AND RELIGION

Why do so many people who turn to God for help with their weight wind up failing?

When you pray to God and he still doesn't remove your food problem, it's not that God isn't listening—it's that there are other steps you need to take in order to let God help you. Those steps are exactly what this book is about. And the first step is to understand what the *real* problem is.

WHAT REALLY WORKS

I've already told you, "It's not about the food," and you may even agree with that, to some extent. But you still may be wondering, "What does she mean?" And "If it isn't about the food, what *is* it about?"

IF YOU FOCUS ON LOSING WEIGHT OR CONTROLLING FOOD, YOU'LL NEVER LOSE WEIGHT OR GET CONTROL OF FOOD.

It's so easy to believe that the food and the weight are the problem and that losing weight and stopping your overeating is the solution. But if you focus on losing weight or controlling food, you'll never lose weight or get control of food. It's counterintuitive, I know. But after being on this road for decades and helping hundreds of others along the way, it's my experience nonetheless.

Being overweight is a symptom of overeating. And overeating is a symptom of what's eating *you*.

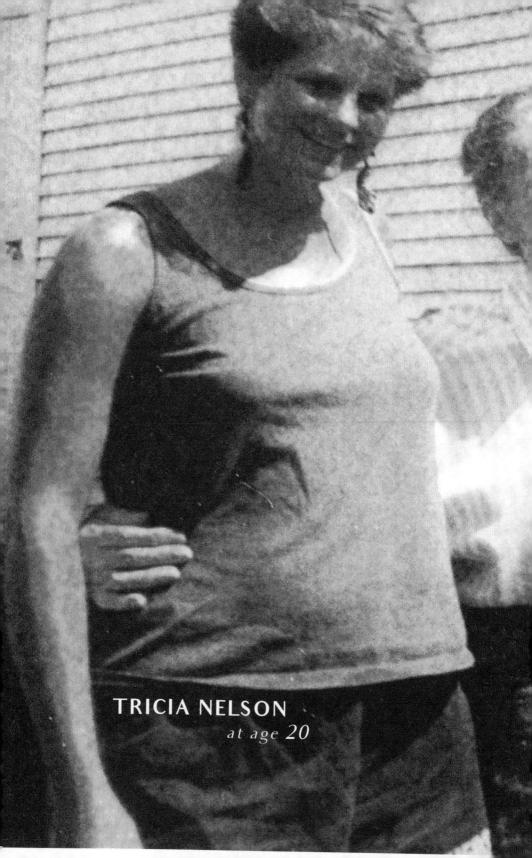

TRICIA NELSON
at age 20

why WE EAT

Let's take a look at a common scenario. Sarah, aged forty, has a family, holds a job outside the home, and is active in her community.

Her typical day looks like this:

6:30 a.m. Her alarm rings; she hits the snooze button twice and finally gets up, with only six hours of sleep. She's running late for work but has to get the kids ready for school, so she skips breakfast and heads to the office.

8:55 a.m. Sarah grabs half a doughnut and some coffee from the office kitchen.

9:00 a.m.–6:00 p.m. Sarah spends her day at work meeting deadlines and keeping appointments. Dealing with an ornery client, she has to work right through lunch.

6:00 p.m. Sarah leaves work and picks up the kids from school, then picks up groceries to make dinner.

7:00 p.m. Sarah gets home to find a long list of phone calls to return and tweets and Facebook posts to answer. She makes dinner, but since she has a committee meeting tonight, she doesn't have any time to sit and eat with her family. Instead, she grabs a few bites standing over the sink and tells herself she'll eat later, when she gets home from the meeting. And does she ever.

9:30 p.m. Sarah gets home, puts the kids to bed, and checks some more office emails. She feels stressed, exhausted and FAMISHED.

10:00 p.m. Although she's tired and needs to go to bed, Sarah heads down to the kitchen instead and opens the refrigerator. She'll just eat a small bowl of cereal to help her relax.

That one bowl turns into three . . . followed by a few slices of bread and some melted cheese . . . then some cinnamon toast, then two bowls of ice cream, and the rest of the bag of chocolate chips she was saving for the cookies she was going to make for her son's soccer meet.

Any of this sound familiar? It's a common syndrome and one that's hard to stop.

Here's how it happens: The next day, Sarah wakes up and vows to eat very little to "make up for" the damage of the night before. She does well with this plan until three in the afternoon, when at last her resolve is no match for her physical hunger and emotional stress, and she can't help but repeat the same cycle all over again. And so she does.

The fact is, our bodies need proper nourishment. The problem is, we emotional eaters don't know the difference between eating because our bodies actually need food to function, and eating because we *feel* hungry but are eating for a completely different reason. This makes it close to impossible to tell the difference between physical hunger and emotional hunger.

WHAT CAUSES "REAL" HUNGER?

While the mechanics of physical hunger are no doubt interesting, they are of only limited use to the chronic emotional eater. My experience is that the emotional eater's solution lies primarily in the emotional and spiritual realm. Still, we do need a rudimentary understanding of how our bodies respond to the physical condition of hunger.

Hunger starts when certain nutrients are missing from the bloodstream. A message goes to the hunger center in our brain, via the "hunger hormone" known as *ghrelin*, which is released from our gut when we're low on nutrients and need to fuel up. Ghrelin, discovered only in 1996, is a complex hormone that controls not only appetite but also the storage of fat. Our bodies also release it in response to stress, stimulating our tendency to stress-eat. When our blood has enough of the needed nutrients, our hunger center stops getting ghrelin signals, and we no longer feel hungry.

At least, that's the way it's *supposed* to work.

Unfortunately, ghrelin is also released when we see an attractive slice of cake, so it's not a particularly discriminating hormone!

Now, if you're an emotional eater, you don't even need the potent combo of ghrelin and cake to feel hungry. Your hunger center may never even need to send a signal that your body needs nutrients. Because if you're one of the many people who use food to self-anesthetize—to deal with stress, fear, exhaustion, and loneliness—your body may have incorporated a tendency to feel hungry as part of your physiology. *And it may also stop getting the message when you're full.*

That means you've trained your body to respond to a negative state by yelling, "Feed me!"

Getting back to Sarah's example, if you haven't eaten all day, your body may be expressing a real and valid hunger. But also, you may have caused imbalances in your body by your erratic eating behavior, thus making it harder to trust the cues of "hungry" and "full." That's why skipping meals is such a trap and makes it so much harder to differentiate between physical and emotional hunger.

When you eat regularly and don't skip meals, it's easier to understand that when you think you might be hungry only a few hours after eating, what you are feeling probably isn't a need for food, but a need for emotional comfort. You may be searching for a buffer from fear and anxiety. The key is to learn to recognize this and look beyond the knee-jerk reaction of feeling "hungry."

Maybe what you're doing is simply *feeling*.

Emotional eaters are typically afraid of feelings. When we don't have food in our belly, we tend to be more sensitive and more aware of what's going on inside. We're more aware of sadness, loneliness, fear, anger, dread, and other hard-to-manage feelings. Even happy, joyful feelings—which, strangely, are sometimes harder to face than the dark ones—can be overwhelming, especially when we don't feel worthy of feeling good.

When we don't self-anesthetize with excessive eating, we're also more in tune with ourselves and with what our bodies need, even when we don't want to be. For instance, you might know that staying late at work isn't the best way to take care of yourself. But with a few quick trips to the vending machine for chips and candy, you can work straight through till eight or nine.

Without food in our bellies, we might hear that voice that says, "You're doing too much; stop working now." If our senses aren't dulled from snacking throughout the day, we might recognize that we're feeling lonely and disconnected. All kinds of emotions surface when our bellies aren't full.

Emotions are difficult for emotional eaters. We tend to avoid them like the plague. Our need to avoid emotions is often what prompts our confusion about hunger sensations. It's why we blindly believe our bodies and minds when we think we're hungry, without doing a little detective work. This puts us in a position to be eating all the time and never having peace around food.

ALL KINDS OF EMOTIONS SURFACE WHEN OUR BELLIES AREN'T FULL.

Of course, if you're reading this book, you've already tried various methods hoping to make peace with food, but none of them have worked. You may even have asked yourself, *Why can't I stop? Why am I doing this? What is wrong with me?*

The answer lies in something I call the PEP formula.

WHAT IS PEP?

The concept of PEP is based on the theory that emotional eaters eat as an answer to deeper problems—which is why just stopping and "getting over it" is impossible. The underlying problems are still there.

Most people try to stop overeating because of what the excess weight and torture of the food obsession is doing **to** them. But the real key to stopping the madness is to look more closely at what food is doing *for* them.

You see, it's impossible to stop any addiction without first realizing that the addiction serves an emotional function. The addictive behavior "solves" a problem, albeit in a twisted way that doesn't really solve anything.

What problem does the addictive eating solve? It serves as a means of anesthetizing three primary emotions: pain, fear, and guilt. So we use food as . . .

- **P** – Painkiller (to relieve pain)
- **E** – Escape (to escape fear)
- **P** – Punishment (to treat guilt)

THE **"PEP"** FORMULA

	ADDICTION AS A	DRIVING EMOTION
P	PAINKILLER	PAIN
E	ESCAPE	FEAR
P	PUNISHMENT	GUILT

PAIN

No matter how happy we seem or how functional our lives appear to be on the outside, we emotional eaters have underlying pain that we try to deaden with food. When we eat, we enter a numb state where we can't feel much of anything. In fact, many emotional eaters gravitate toward heavy, calorie-rich "comfort foods" (the name says it all, doesn't it?) because they are the most effective means of deadening our uncomfortable emotions.

That's why the sugary, starchy, fatty foods do the trick. They make us feel full (stuffed) and sedated, so our binge momentarily lets us forget our troubles. This is why we are rarely drawn to binge on lighter, more watery foods. Think about it: how often have you binged on *salad*?

ESCAPE

The next thing emotional eaters use food addiction for is as an escape. Like all addicts, we emotional eaters typically have a part of us that just doesn't want to deal. And we often have so much fear that we feel as though we just can't cope. Life seems overwhelming, scary, and just too much for us to face day in and day out. We feel tired of being a "good boy" or "good girl," doing things right or being on top of our game. There's a part of us that just feels like checking out.

Of course, everyone needs to escape sometimes. Everyone has stress in their lives, and everyone needs to get away from that stress. That's why we take vacations! It's also why we go to movies or read books or do whatever kind of

we like to do, physical and otherwise. These are all healthy ways to
e pressures and rigors of life.

fferent about emotional eaters is that we pervert this normal human
to the point that we crave escape and have a strong aversion to reality.

WE DON'T WANT TO DEAL WITH REALITY, WITH RESPONSIBILITIES, WITH *FEELINGS.*

As you will learn in the chapter Anatomy of the Emotional Eater®, emotional eaters are abnormally fearful. No matter what is going on, life seems harder for us than for the average person. We don't want to deal with reality, with responsibilities, with feelings. We would much rather bury our heads in the sand. And food helps us do that.

Imagine someone coming home at the end of the day after putting in a full, stressful day dealing with the realities of work. They walk in, and there are bills, chores, and mouths to feed. It feels like too much. Then they open the refrigerator and eat for hours because it quells their stress, quiets their mind, and helps them shut out the world and all its demands.

Why does an emotional eater turn to food instead of being truly present with family and friends? For one thing, these are often some of the aspects of reality that emotional eaters feel the need to escape from! Sometimes, we don't want to be "good" and exercise. We're tired and stressed, and *we want to be left alone.* We don't want to deal with people—spouse and kids included.

For an emotional eater, food provides the quickest, easiest escape from stress and fear.

PUNISHMENT
Imagine baking a batch of cookies, opening a pint of Häagen-Dazs, and sitting down in front of the TV for a relaxing evening. It might feel like bliss: time to yourself and nothing to do but enjoy it. It's the perfect escape from the cares (read *fears*) of the day. In fact, you're so blissed out, you forget to stop eating. You finish everything and probably return to the kitchen for something more. (Gotta have something salty after all those sweets!)

But the next morning, after the goodies are gone, you're left with self-loathing, a bloated body, and a strong desire to hide from other people.

Most of us are raised to see food as a reward. We grow up hearing things such as "Eat all your vegetables and you can have dessert." And we carry this into our adult lives: after a long day at work, we come home and reward ourselves with our favorite snack, which turns into a binge.

What emotional eaters may not see is the ugly flip side to that "reward." The clothes that don't fit, the acne from the greasy foods, the shame over our bodies, the gorgeous days spent hiding indoors, the embarrassment and disgust over not being able to control our eating—unlike everyone else.

These, and so many other negative factors that accompany emotional eating, are forms of self-punishment and self-sabotage. But most of us don't really connect the dots between our penchant for food and our self-destructive eating habits. The fact is that deep down in every food addict is a built-in desire for punishment, self-sabotage, and destruction. It usually comes from a deep-seated sense of worthlessness, a feeling we got from our early childhood. Somehow, somewhere deep inside, is the belief that we're bad, we're stupid, we're ugly, and we deserve to be punished. So we punish ourselves by bingeing and then hating ourselves afterward.

As a result, what may have started out feeling like a reward is actually the worst form of punishment an emotional eater could ever endure. And yet, we do endure it, over and over and over again—sometimes for a lifetime.

To be free of emotional eating, you must address the hidden problems that cause it: the underlying pain that you use food to numb, the fears that make you want to escape, and the guilt you harbor inside that makes you believe you deserve to be punished.

When you address these hidden, underlying causes, they will no longer drive you to overeat.

In the next chapter, you'll learn about the personality traits that govern our reactions to life and end up creating the pain, fear, and guilt that drive our overeating.

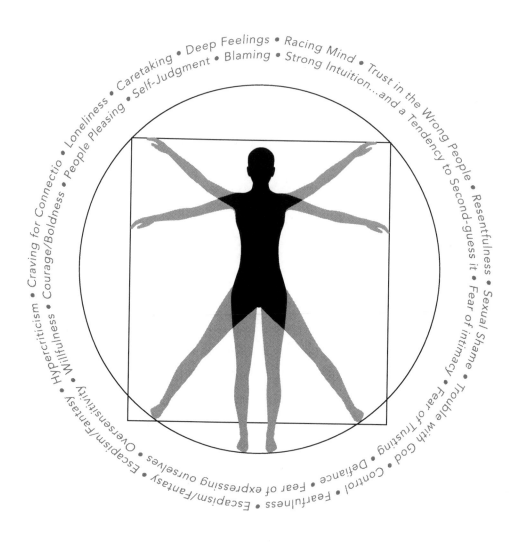

chapter 4

anatomy of the
EMOTIONAL
eater®

The emotional eater is a special breed. Our feelings, thought patterns, and reactions are different, and they are more pronounced than those of other people. Coming to understand this can give tremendous relief to those of us who have spent our lives wondering, "What is wrong with me?"

We already know we aren't like others around us. We compare ourselves and always seem to come up short. We are sure that our friends and family members have it "going on." They are self-assured, smart, witty, and confident. And the more we beat on ourselves for not being that way, the worse we feel—and the more we turn to food for solace. It's a vicious cycle, and we don't know how to stop it or even how it started.

So what is the difference between an emotional eater and a "normal" person? Having spent decades working with emotional eaters and overcoming my own issues as well, I have come to identify a particular list of characteristics that, taken together, begin to form a personality profile of the emotional eater. Other people also have many of these traits—after all, these are human qualities. But emotional eaters have a greater number of these qualities and experience them more intensely than the average person. That's why I refer to this set of traits as the Anatomy of the Emotional Eater®.

I'm not assuming that you will identify (or even *should* identify) with every one of these qualities. Some of them may truly not fit you. But be aware that you may have some of these qualities without recognizing it, because overeating has made you blind to them.

Consider our own physical anatomy as an analogy. You have lots of systems that operate in your body without your conscious direction or knowledge, yet they still serve a vital function. Similarly, you may not identify with some of the following characteristics, yet they may still be an integral part of how you live and react to life.

EMOTIONAL EATERS HAVE A LIVING PROBLEM, NOT AN EATING PROBLEM.

Understanding the traits that make you tick will help you understand just how true it is that *food is not the problem*. This condition has little to do with food, and much to do with how we live our lives, and the stress and chaos that we create for ourselves, based on these traits. As Roy often says, "You don't have an eating problem; you have a living problem."

THE PROFILE

If you suspect you're an emotional eater, you will likely find yourself saying, "Check, check, check," as you recognize the traits that aptly describe you.

DEEP FEELINGS

Emotional eaters are, well, emotional! We feel more deeply than the average person. When we hear sad news, it hits us hard. When people we love are hurting, we hurt, too. When we love, we love deeply, and when we hate, we hate vehemently. Life often feels like an emotional roller-coaster ride, so food becomes a means of balancing out the highs and lows. We are emotionally absorbent, so everything seems to hurt. And we turn to food to dull the ache.

OVERSENSITIVITY

Do you get a lot of comments such as "You're so sensitive," or "You wear your heart on your sleeve"? You might think you're somehow wrong or bad because of it. Well, guess again. You're not. You're just sensitive. I tend to believe that as emotional eaters, we were born this way, but experiencing pain in our childhood can make us extra sensitive, as well. Of course, growing up with a weight problem and feeling different or rejected because of it can also make us feel like a walking pincushion. Being sensitive can be a good thing, but because we haven't had proper tools to deal with our emotions, it has mostly been a liability.

FEARFULNESS

Everyone feels fear. It's a normal human emotion that we all experience. But emotional eaters have an enormous amount of fear: fear of drowning, fear of strangers, fear of monsters under the bed or in the closet, fear of the worst possible things happening. Does any of this sound familiar? Whatever your specific fears happen to be, they erode your sense of well-being and ultimately drive you to eat. When you feel constant, underlying anxiety, you search for something to ease the tension. That's a lot of what all that nibbling is about. We're trying to quell those nameless fears and anxieties that persistently haunt us.

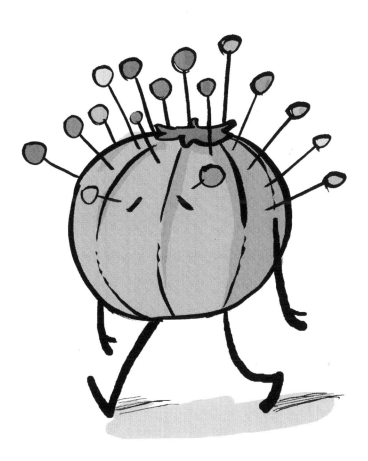

EMOTIONAL EATERS ARE EXTRA SENSITIVE, LIKE A WALKING PINCUSHION.

RACING MIND

Overeaters are *overthinkers*. Our minds race from one thought to another and seem never to stop. Sometimes, we obsess on one thing and then think it to death. Or we worry, which is basically what happens when fear meets the racing mind of an emotional eater. When fear and anxiety persist and we attempt to bury it long enough with food, alcohol, and other painkillers, it can often lead to panic attacks. Our racing minds can also cause insomnia. But even if sleep isn't a problem, sitting still is. We don't like to be idle, and meditation seems out of the question! Most emotional eaters turn to food as their first defense against worry and obsession. Carbohydrates are especially attractive because they provide a serotonin boost that actually helps slow down the mind. It's quite typical for emotional eaters to overeat in order to check out, to quiet our minds so we can relax a bit.

CRAVING FOR CONNECTION

We crave community. We crave being with people. We yearn for that heart-to-heart connection. The crazy thing is, we spend most of our lives keeping any kind of *real* connection at bay—by hiding out in food. Overeating keeps us isolated. It separates us from people by making us feel ashamed and embarrassed. But the truth is that emotional eaters are starving. We are starving for connection and love. We crave it, but alas, we look for it in all the wrong places, ensuring we will never find it. We hook up with emotionally unavailable partners, we work in emotionally toxic environments, and we engage in one-sided friendships with people who are interested only in talking about themselves.

EMOTIONAL EATERS ARE STARVING.

LONELINESS

While emotional eaters have a strong need for connection and love, we also feel as though it is just out of reach. We are plagued by feelings of loneliness. We feel lonely even when we're not literally alone. We can be in a room full of people who are friendly and enjoy being with us, yet we can still feel totally alone and as if we don't fit in. Even when we find a partner later in life, we often don't feel really connected at a deep level. What makes matters worse, when we feel as if we don't fit in or are self-conscious about our weight, we end up avoiding social situations as well as any kind of intimacy. So we essentially treat loneliness with isolation. Makes perfect sense, doesn't it?

Consider the emotional eater's battle cry: "Leave me alone, leave me alone. Can't you see I'm lonely?"

COURAGE/BOLDNESS

Emotional eaters do some very courageous things. We may travel the world, lead a corporation, raise a difficult child, care for ailing parents. But just because we're courageous doesn't mean we are not also afraid. And a lot of times, we're actually trying to compensate for the fear by being bold. People tell us how

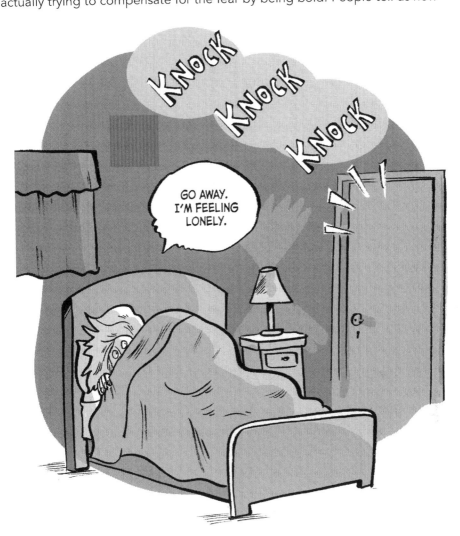

TREATING LONELINESS WITH ISOLATION

© 2017 by Tricia Nelson

courageous we are, and we think, *If you only knew* . . . Because while some fearful people cower and shield themselves from life, others are dealing with the fear by plowing through it, by being outgoing and vivacious. The problem is, we have to use food to back us up. Take the late-night binges, wine-and-steak dinners, and pocketful of candy away from a high-powered, obese executive, and you'll meet a different person. The excessive food and weight have served as the engine for all that vim and vigor.

STRONG INTUITION—AND A TENDENCY TO SECOND-GUESS IT

Emotional eaters are very intuitive. You could say we have that "sixth sense." Everyone has it, but emotional eaters, being deep feelers, have a heightened sensitivity to it. Our intuition protects us when we listen to it. But too often when our intuition gives us the sense that something isn't right, we override it and say, "Oh, no, it's fine." The reason we do this stems mainly from fear and lack of confidence. Our intuition will show us the right thing to do, but we second-guess it and waffle instead of following our hunch. We even argue with our intuition and choose not to take the action it indicates we should take. And this results in more chaos in our lives. How many times have you said, "I had a feeling that guy wasn't any good for me"? Or, "My gut told me this was a bad decision, but I went ahead with it anyway"? Fear and self-doubt cause us to deny our instincts and intuition, but there's another reason, too . . .

WILLFULNESS

Emotional eaters are tremendously willful. And it's not always a bad thing. After all, when we put our mind to something, we get a lot done. But when we insist on having things *our way,* we end up stepping on others' toes and making them angry. We also get upset when they don't do what *we want*. And that strong intuition we have? We often steamroll right over that still, small voice while in hot pursuit of getting things to go our way.

ESCAPISM/FANTASY

Emotional eaters are fantastical thinkers. Because so much in life is scary, we learned from an early age to avoid reality by tripping out with fantasy. In school, we were the daydreamers who were looking out the window instead of paying attention to the teacher. Perhaps we made up elaborate stories about our lives: our family was royalty, a knight in shining armor was on his way to rescue us, we possessed super powers, and so on. The problem is, what started as a harmless children's pastime ends up morphing into a habitual way of thinking as adults. While using food as our buffer from reality, we scripted our life based on how *we wanted it to be*, instead of how it really is. We decided to play by the rules of our own parallel world (where all the rules worked in our favor) while the rest of the world was operating according to reality. When things don't pan out the way we expect, we are frustrated and disappointed and console ourselves with food.

CONTROL

Most emotional eaters have issues with control. We are afraid to be out of control (because that's an uncomfortable feeling), so we try to make things go our way as much as possible. We tend to be know-it-alls, sure that we are smarter than everyone else. We like to tell people what to do, or manipulate them to do it, which makes them feel hurt and resentful, which in turn makes us feel afraid and stressed. After all, we want everyone to like us at the same time they are doing what we say!

SELF-JUDGMENT

As emotional eaters, we give ourselves a hard time. We're not pretty enough, smart enough, good enough; we haven't accomplished enough; we're not doing a good enough job; we're not articulate enough; we're not popular enough; nothing is ever good enough for us. No one is ever as mean to us as we are to ourselves. And to punish ourselves for all the faults and limitations that we perceive in ourselves, we overeat. The irony is that by sabotaging our looks, our productivity, and our effectiveness in relationships and life in general, we end up affirming many of the negative things we believe about ourselves.

HYPERCRITICISM

We emotional eaters aren't just critical of ourselves. We're also hard on other people. We hold others to the same impossible standards as ourselves—and sometimes even higher ones. Other people always get the "spillover" of what we do to ourselves. So when we're harsh, judgmental, and critical of ourselves, we are harsh, judgmental, and critical of others. But this stubborn habit makes us feel guilty and perpetuates the need to punish ourselves with food.

RESENTFULNESS

The evil twin of people pleasing is resentment. Because if you're out there working twenty hours more than everybody else in the office, you expect something in return. You're trying to please others, because you want them to validate you. But when you don't get the validation you seek, you get mad. Just to be clear, you're not trying to please people because you want them to be happy; you're doing it because you want them to express their appreciation and approval of you. But they never do—at least, not in the way you had planned. So you burn with resentment. Emotional eaters typically have something stuck in their craw, without even realizing it.

BLAMING

I hate to say it, but as emotional eaters we are superb blamers. After all, it's so easy to do, and it feels so good—in the moment. As emotional eaters, we don't like to feel, let alone take responsibility for our uncomfortable feelings, so we look for someone or something to blame. It's not a conscious thing. Indeed, it's quite unconscious, but it's a deeply ingrained habit. As my husband, Roy Nelson, says, "If other people are our problem, we're screwed—there are too many of them and we can't possibly change them all!" So long as we blame anyone else for how we feel, we never can get to the true cause of why we feel bad. We will be perpetually unhappy. Of course, when we hold on to the victim narrative, we have a perfect excuse for overeating, every time.

PEOPLE PLEASING

It's been said of those with "people-pleasing" tendencies that if you put a hundred people in a room, and ninety-nine of them like us and one doesn't, you will invariably find us over there with the one-hundredth person, trying to get them to like us, instead of just enjoying the ninety-nine who already do! The fact is, it drives most emotional eaters crazy if somebody doesn't like them. The reason is because emotional eaters seek validation from others instead of from themselves. Typically, this results from low self-esteem. That's why emotional eaters tend to be such great workers: because they go above and beyond the call of duty to make sure they get every drop of praise they can from their boss and coworkers.

FEAR OF EXPRESSING OURSELVES

We're afraid to express what we think or feel, and we eat to cover up those feelings that we were afraid to express. I have an expression: "Share it or wear it." That doesn't mean going around telling everybody how you really feel about them (especially when it's not too nice). But when something bothers you, you've got to speak up about it. Emotional eaters bottle up their emotions, and they use food to do it. It's called *stuffing your feelings.* Which reminds me of another favorite expression: "Say it or stuff it."

SEXUAL SHAME

It's very common for emotional eaters and people with eating disorders to have experienced sexual abuse in their past. This is often what triggered our food problems in the first place. In an effort to bury this pain and shame and to

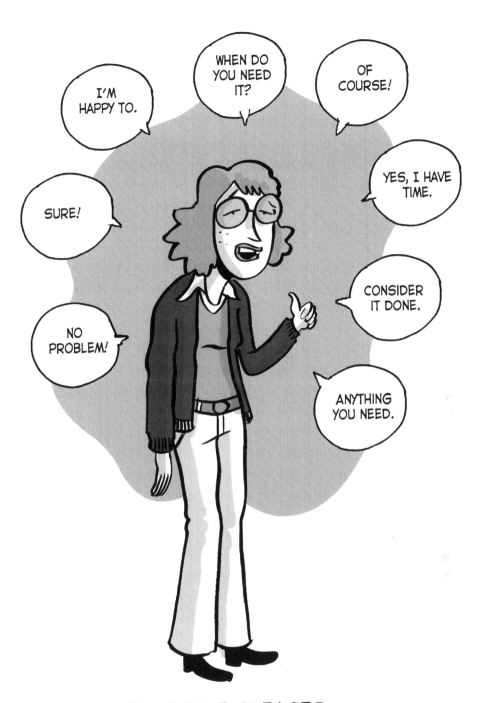

THE PEOPLE PLEASER

protect ourselves from further abuse, we have hidden behind mounds of food and fat. The shame we carry about our bodies and our sexual behavior (be it masturbation, porn, promiscuity, or asexuality) continues to haunt us and make us feel unworthy of love. Our shame makes us feel separate from others.

FEAR OF INTIMACY

Fear of intimacy is practically universal for emotional eaters. We carry so much shame and doubt about our bodies and our intrinsic worth that getting close to someone, sexually or not, can be a frightening prospect. We are afraid to let down our guard and let people see who we really are. We are sure that if anyone really knew us, they would reject us. So we keep our guard up and don't allow anyone in.

CARETAKING

Emotional eaters are great caretakers—again, often stemming from childhood patterns. Being sensitive to others' pain and being people pleasers makes us naturally assume the role of caretaker in our family, our marriage, and our job. Ever notice how the health-care industry, which is all about caring for others, is full of obese nurses? This is because of the extreme stress and long hours of this type of work, and because nurses are so busy taking care of others that they neglect to take care of themselves. Another tendency for emotional eaters is to hook up with alcoholics. They fit hand in glove: the alcoholic is busy making messes and the overeater is busy cleaning up the messes.

TROUBLE WITH GOD

Many of us were fed a heavy dose of religion when we were growing up. (That's a nicer way of saying we had it shoved down our throats.) You may have been taught about a vengeful, punishing God, and frankly, it scared you. As Roy says, "With a God like that, who needed a devil?" (But of course, they threw in a devil, anyway!) Being supersensitive and deep-feeling children, we took these heavy-handed messages about God, our sinful nature, and the likelihood that we were going to hell pretty hard. At some point, it was just too much. We'd had enough. So we rejected the notion of God that we had learned, and often turned our back on religion. Some of us became atheists, but most of us were simply bitter and lost. Many of us wanted the comfort of believing in God but were conflicted about the messages we had learned, and wondered whether we could ever find solace in a higher power. To make matters worse, we asked God to remove our overeating problem, and when nothing improved, we wondered whether God was listening or even cared.

FEAR OF TRUSTING

Emotional eaters are afraid to trust. We typically had situations in our past where we trusted someone and that trust was betrayed. Perhaps it was an alcoholic parent or an inappropriate relative, teacher, or clergy member who took advantage of our vulnerability. At that point, our young mind made the decision that trusting *anyone* was a bad idea, a prescription for disappointment. So as adults, we are habitually leery of people who are nice to us, and wonder whether they have ulterior motives. We have built a wall around our heart, and we don't let it down easily, if ever. This causes tension in our relationships and often prevents us from being able to experience true intimacy of any kind.

TRUST IN THE WRONG PEOPLE

The irony is that emotional eaters who are afraid to trust are routinely taken in by the wrong people. (We have been burned all those times, and we still never see it coming.) The truth is that our very fear of trusting causes us to attract people who are not trustworthy. When our hearts are closed, we end up being strangers to ourselves. When we don't know ourselves, we can't know others, can't detect their motives and intentions. So we are easily deluded and get hurt all over again.

> **OUR VERY FEAR OF TRUSTING CAUSES US TO ATTRACT PEOPLE WHO ARE NOT TRUSTWORTHY.**

DEFIANCE

Emotional eaters don't like to be told what to do, plain and simple. And we don't like rules. So no matter how compliant we appear on the outside (because, as people pleasers, we don't want to make anyone mad), just below the surface we have a strong defiant streak. We often give people in authority a terrible time. Whether with our parents, a teacher, or a boss, our knee-jerk reaction is always "Don't tell me what to do!" or, echoing Sinatra, "I'll do it my way." (You may even notice those thoughts coming up as you read this book.) Incidentally, this is one of the problems with prescribed diets: we want someone to tell us what to eat, but ultimately we're bound to rebel!

WHY THE PROFILE MATTERS

This list of traits may be a bit overwhelming to read, but I'm hoping you also found it comforting.

Here's what I believe is most important about this information:

1. **It confirms that you are not alone.**

   These traits and ways of thinking, with a few variations, are common to every emotional eater's experience. So you no longer have to assume you're the "only one" who thinks this way or does these things. There are millions of emotional eaters who think and act just like you. Later on, I'll show you how to be in contact and community with them so you will be further comforted to find that not only are you not alone, but you are also supported in making healing changes.

2. **It shows you that having these qualities is not your fault.**

   God knows you don't need another reason to beat yourself up! These traits are not your fault, nor are they all bad. And they can be modified and tempered to work for you instead of against you. Every personality trait that you have is a result of living in the environment where you were raised; they were adaptive tools you used as a means of self-protection. But some of them have outgrown their usefulness to you. The "7 Simple Steps" outlined in the next several chapters are geared toward helping you build new coping tools so it will be easier to loosen your grip on the old, outworn ones.

3. **It's another reminder that food is not the problem.**

   Remember, emotional eaters have a living problem, not an eating problem. The obsession with food and weight is a symptom of the stress and pain we create when we have (and act on) certain personality traits. So if you want to end emotional eating, you must focus far more on tempering these traits than on what you should eat and how many calories you should burn.

4. **These qualities have an upside and a downside.**

   Sure, many of these traits land us in hot water over and over again, but there's often an upside. For instance, take being fearful. Fear can stop us in our tracks and make us not follow through on pursuing a dream, such as a career we've always wanted. But fear can also protect us. When friends invite us to go hiking in the mountains but they don't seem to have thought it through, we feel dubious and stay home. Turns out that because they didn't have a map and compass, our friends got lost and two of them experienced frostbite. So in that case, fear, manifested as caution, was a good thing!

The key is to become better acquainted with who we are and what makes us tick, so we can live in the solution and sidestep the traps that our thoughts and behaviors can sometimes set for us.

Download your AEE worksheet to begin healing your three most pronounced traits at www.healyourhungerbook.com.

PART 2

THE PATH

7 simple steps TO END EMOTIONAL *eating now*

"THE SEVEN C'S FOR HEALING"

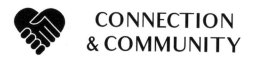
CONNECTION & COMMUNITY

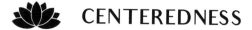
CENTEREDNESS

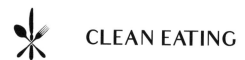
CLEAN EATING

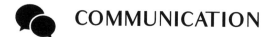
COMMUNICATION

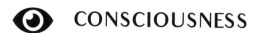
CONSCIOUSNESS

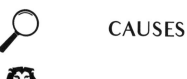
CAUSES

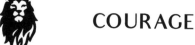
COURAGE

THE SEVEN C'S FOR HEALING

I have to be honest here. Writing this book was a real challenge, because there are so many layers to healing emotional eating. And if I tried to fit everything I've learned into this book, it would be a tome too big to lift, and you'd never bother reading it.

There is no silver-bullet answer to the food and weight-loss conundrum. That's what makes it a conundrum! But I truly believe that the next several chapters will get you to the heart of why you overeat, and show you how to stop.

But be forewarned: these aren't going to be easy steps. Simple? Yes. Easy? Not really.

And while at times it may seem as if what you're reading has nothing to do with food and weight, please trust me—it does.

I call these steps "The Seven C's for Healing."

Each of these elements is powerful on its own. But to fully heal the underlying issues that drive our food addiction, and be completely free of the compulsion to eat self-destructively, you will need *all of them* in your life.

The next seven chapters will lay out exactly what you need in order to transform your relationship with food. Each chapter will focus on one of the vital aspects of healing and why it is important.

I'm not saying this is the only way. But in my experience, not only is addressing the underlying causes the most direct route to healing emotional eating, but it also ensures that you'll be happy when you do. Those who struggle with weight believe "I'll be happy when I'm thin." But "I'll be thin when I'm happy" is more accurate. These seven simple steps can make that happen.

One more thing: I don't want you ever to feel overwhelmed or alone with this information. For that reason, I want to remind you that additional support is available if you need it.

**To access additional information and support
go to www.healyourhungerbook.com.**

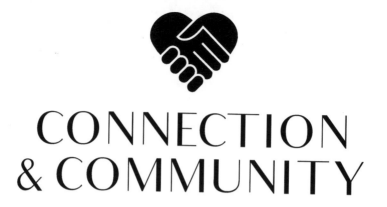

CONNECTION & COMMUNITY

 CENTEREDNESS

 CLEAN EATING

 COMMUNICATION

 CONSCIOUSNESS

 CAUSES

 COURAGE

chapter 5

CONNECTION
& *community*

One of the deepest feelings that we numb through emotional eating is the feeling of disconnection from the people around us—even those we're supposed to feel close to.

Why does this happen? Well, some of the traits I talked about in Anatomy of the Emotional Eater® certainly contribute. Being overly sensitive, fearful, judgmental; overthinking everything (such as others' comments); having a need to control others; being resentful, ashamed of our bodies, and afraid of trusting people—all these aspects of our personality leave us feeling isolated and disconnected from others. In the back of our mind we think, *If people really knew me, they wouldn't like me or accept me.*

IN THE BACK OF OUR MIND WE THINK, *IF PEOPLE REALLY KNEW ME, THEY WOULDN'T LIKE ME OR ACCEPT ME.*

Because the fear and the untrue belief that we are bad and unlovable is so deeply rooted within our psyches, we actually prove this to be true time and time again. Fearing that we will be rejected, we tend to be guarded, defensive, and hesitant to express our authentic selves, which ensures that people can never get to know us or embrace who we really are.

So we fulfill our fear of being unlovable.

Our desperate need for approval makes us overcompensate for our insecurities by being outgoing, helpful, and overly friendly. But people can sense our neediness, and it's a turnoff. So once again, we have successfully proved what we feared was true: that we aren't loveable after all.

The irony is that we crave intimacy more than anything else in the world and, at the same, deeply fear it. We reject those who want to be close to us (often treating them badly), and we are attracted to those who are incapable of being close. You may recognize them as "emotionally unavailable."

Either way, the result is the same: we feel achingly lonely and disconnected. And to comfort ourselves, we eat. But instead of helping us feel better, the food just fuels our unhappiness and sense of isolation and rejection.

Does this sound at all familiar?

Connecting with others, with ourselves, and with God is crucial to breaking the destructive cycle of emotional eating. Plain and simple, no one can overcome emotional eating unless they connect at the heart level with one or more people who understand them and can truly care about them.

As Roy often says, "I needed someone who understood and cared. I often found people who understood but didn't care, or people who cared but didn't understand, but I needed someone who could both understand and care before I was able to heal."

The reason we must have this connection is simple: without connection, without solving that terrible sense of isolation we feel, we remain trapped inside ourselves, where we will eventually implode under the weight of unexpressed thoughts and feelings.

But while we desperately need to reach outside ourselves, our ego and pride are so strong that we fight fiercely for our right to "go it alone." If food addicts could get away with it, they would never humble themselves to the point of needing anything from anyone.

This is the dilemma we face. On the one hand, we desperately crave and seek love and connection; on the other, we reject that love in favor of the "safety" of isolation.

I understand how desperate and painful it is to feel so alone. I was always plagued with this feeling until I began to heal. But being a food addict provides a hidden blessing: *it forces us to reach out for help.* The pain of our condition drives us to reach outside ourselves and make that connection.

If we want to heal, we can't go it alone. And connecting with those who understand and care is what creates the environment for healing.

Believe it or not, those most likely to understand and care about your struggles are not your family and friends. People you are closest to have usually been "in the fire" with you to one degree or another. They have been sick with worry; they've been hurt; they've had their hearts broken. They are often resentful, angry, and fed up. After all, how many times have you gone on a diet and declared that you're finally going to lose that weight "for good"? So they cheer you on and get excited about your progress—until the day that they walk in the door and see you eating half a tray of fudge right before their eyes. For the next several days, they witness you giving up and giving in, and your subsequent descent into depression, hostility, and self-loathing. Needless to say, your family members may not have the love and understanding you need them to have. More importantly, even if they want to support you through a new attempt at recovery, they really can't unless they've been in your shoes.

It's really hard for family and friends to understand why you sabotage your relationships and your life the way you do. As much as they want to understand the pain and anguish you feel when you are on a diet and don't have your food fix, they can't. And then when you do get your "fix" and spin out of control, they can't understand that, either. So there is an obvious disconnection there. They want to understand, but for someone who has never felt powerless over a doughnut, how could they?

Some well-meaning family, friends, or even doctors or therapists may say, "Why don't you try to moderate and start being more physically active?" When people tell us this, it's a clear indication that they don't understand our predicament—that we can't just moderate or exercise more, or else we would have done it long ago—and that the problem is deeper than that. Just know that when people make comments that are unhelpful, it's only because they truly don't understand. How lucky they are!

The greatest sense of connection you will feel is when you talk to someone who has experienced what you are going through and has come to the other side.

For example, I didn't empathize with people who had a parent die of cancer, until my father died of cancer in 2001. Suddenly, I had this huge place in my heart for people who were going through that awful experience or had been through it. I knew exactly how they felt: the grief, sense of helplessness, and horror of watching a healthy, vibrant loved one deteriorate before their eyes. All of a sudden, I felt *connected* with those who had similar experiences. I wanted to help them, support them, and let them know that the grief does lessen with time. When I did reach out, there was an automatic bond between us. This is the same type of bond that emotional eaters feel when they can talk to someone else who understands their struggles and can offer a solution.

The problem with some support groups for people with food issues is that it's easy to get stuck in a pattern of talking about the problem without actively seeking a solution. That can get old pretty fast. There are eating-disorder communities where people are mired in their eating disorder and there isn't a lot of hope. Some anorexics and bulimics have actually learned new eating-disorder tricks from such communities! So while it's comforting to identify with those who have had similar experiences, don't just stop there. The best thing to do is connect with people who are really interested in healing their problem, not just dwelling on it.

Where can we find people to connect with? The *Heal Your Hunger* community is a place you can start. I created this safe space for emotional eaters to connect immediately with others who are struggling and who want to heal. This helps diminish the feeling that you are all alone in your struggles, and gives you support when you need it most: as you set out on your path to healing.

When you connect with emotional eaters who are also hurting and seeking a solution, your heart will be filled with love. You will be reminded of how widespread this condition is and how vital it is that we join forces in overcoming it. The feeling is electric and will feed your soul in a way that no amount of food possibly could.

COMMUNITY

In the book Connected: *The Surprising Power of Our Social Networks and How They Shape Our Lives—How Your Friends' Friends' Friends Affect Everything You Feel, Think, and Do,* Harvard researchers Nicholas Christakis and James Fowler proved that you have a 57 percent greater risk of becoming obese if your friend becomes obese.

They also discovered that this same powerful influence can work in the opposite direction. When a friend or family member loses weight, it influences others around them to lose weight, as well.

So your friends will negatively or positively affect your weight. And you will affect theirs. It makes sense, doesn't it? Obesity begets obesity, and healthy habits beget healthy habits.

It's the same with exercise, too. If you're around people who don't value getting out of the house and walking, jogging, or playing Frisbee, chances are, you're going to lose interest in these things, too. Then again, maybe *you're* the one influencing them to stay on the couch!

Does this mean you ditch your obese friends? No, but if you want to overcome emotional eating, you do need to consider who you hang out with and what activities you engage in when you're together. For instance, instead of meeting for lunch, suggest that you meet for tea or a walk in the botanical garden or at the art museum. This will redirect your time together so it isn't focused on food.

This is one reason why becoming engaged in a community of emotional eaters who are practicing healthy habits in every area of their lives is essential. You could have a 57 percent easier time abstaining from emotional eating just by doing this! But there are other reasons, too.

I have learned, both from personal experience and from over twenty-eight years of helping people overcome their addictions, that if you're an emotional eater, there is nothing more healing than the feeling that there is a place where you truly belong, where you are truly understood.

This is probably because, for as long as most of us can remember, we emotional eaters have been plagued with a sense that we *don't* belong. A lot of us tend to feel as if we were born into the wrong family, or were dropped onto this planet by an alien ship. We're not sure why, but we just don't "fit in."

> **WE EMOTIONAL EATERS HAVE BEEN PLAGUED WITH A SENSE THAT WE DON'T BELONG.**

When we look at the people around us, it seems that they all got the playbook for this thing called life, but for some reason, we didn't get our copy. We see people laughing and having fun, and instead of joining in, we sit on the sidelines, nervously wondering whether they're laughing at us, or whether we will be rejected if we try to join in.

It can sometimes feel as if there were a wall between us and other people. We may have friends, we may form relationships, and, of course, most of us have family members we can talk and interact with (at least, occasionally). But no matter how many people accept us, we still feel as if we were somehow strange or different from the rest of the world. Even if we look as though we fit in, we still tend to feel awkward and out of place. No matter what's going on in our lives, it seems we can't shake the feeling that we don't quite belong.

How many times have you been at a party or among a group of people at dinner and looked around thinking, *no one understands me*, or *I'm not like these people?* Addicts in general have an amazing capacity for feeling lonely even in a room filled with people.

Community isn't just about being with people. It's about being with people you can connect with—people with whom you feel safe being *yourself.* Without the comfort of knowing there is a place where we belong, with people who understand us, food will remain one of the only comforts we feel we can rely on.

After all, how many times have you thought to yourself, *food is the only thing I can count on; it's always there for me?* While it's generally true that food is always available when the going gets tough, if you look a little closer, food is not your friend. Food seduces us into believing that it is our only friend, but then it turns on us and makes us feel more alone than ever.

We need to find community with people who can give us true support, not the *illusion* of support that we relied on food to give us. If we want to overcome emotional eating, the best kind of community will be with *other emotional eaters.* Belonging to a bridge club will not provide the same sense of community as being among other self-admitted emotional eaters and food addicts. Like connecting at the heart level with someone who has been in your shoes, community happens when you are engaging with others who have the same problem as you, with whom you can share that most personal, private part of your life.

Let's look at all the ways that belonging to a community of people who understand you as an emotional eater can help you:

1. The problem that was always a dark secret can finally be brought into the open and discussed freely.

2. You have people you can turn to when you're struggling with food and with life.

3. You feel accepted unconditionally.

4. You can reciprocate by helping others who need support.

We emotional eaters resist having community, because we judge ourselves, our weight, and how we look, talk, and act. And we figure we'll embarrass ourselves or be ridiculed if we let others know us. We figure that our fundamental flaws might be accidentally exposed if we are around others for too long.

The neatest thing about being part of a community of people who have these very same fears is that there is nothing you can't talk about. We've all done and thought virtually the same things, all the while thinking we're the only ones, so it becomes almost funny to hear someone else speak the same crazy ideas that run through your own mind!

Years ago I recorded and posted a "garbage eating" video on YouTube. It's about the shame and humiliation of an old habit: fetching food from the garbage that I had thrown out in a fit of disgust after a binge. By now it has received many thousands of hits because, for binge eaters, this is a fairly common experience. Yet someone who wouldn't binge until stuffed, let alone eat food from the garbage, could not possibly know what that experience is like or why we do it. That's why it helps emotional eaters to find camaraderie with others who share the same rather bizarre experience around obsession with food. Just knowing that someone out there is going through the same thing we are diminishes the hidden shame and degradation we have lived with for way too long.

The fact that we've all been there gives us a level of compassion and acceptance that someone who hasn't been in our shoes cannot possibly have. And imagine the sense of camaraderie that comes with discussing your deepest fears with those who have been plagued by the very same fears and have found a way to overcome them!

This notion of communing with others who struggle with food and weight isn't new. It's how Weight Watchers became so successful.

Twelve-step programs are also based on this principle of communing with other addicts. In fact, Alcoholics Anonymous is the most successful treatment for alcoholism known to mankind. Many people with food addiction have found much identification, comfort, and healing in the various twelve-step programs that deal with food addiction.

But if you've ever been involved in a twelve-step program for food issues, yet continued to struggle, you may be thinking, "That form of community didn't work for me." I get that, because that was my experience, too.

My path started in the twelve-step rooms, but when it came to overeating, I couldn't stop no matter how many meetings I attended. While I will be forever grateful for the education I got on the progression of food addiction—which is very similar to the progression with alcohol for the alcoholic—this program didn't have the level of community I craved, or the deeper healing I required in order to have lasting freedom from my obsession with food.

By this, I mean that I needed more guidance and fellowship than a one-hour meeting and a food sponsor could give me. When everyone would disperse at the end of the meeting, I was left needing more. I craved more interaction and more support. Plagued by a sense of loneliness, I needed more emotional and spiritual nourishment than the meetings provided. I still had a big, gaping hole in my soul. My craving for love and truth ran deep. If I wasn't fed by these meetings, sooner or later I would have to turn back again to food, which I did.

I needed to be shown new coping skills to avoid falling back on the old ones that didn't work. It was vitally important that I be supported in exploring new aspects of my personality that would help diminish stress and create healthier relationships. I had to be challenged to address and walk through my fears so that I was no longer in bondage to them. And every change I made directly affected my relationship with food.

If you're an emotional eater, chances are that to realize ongoing healing, you're going to need a community of emotional eaters focused on a real solution. You must have people you can relate with, who can illuminate a clear path by which you can cope with the ups and downs of life without the crutch of excess food. Whether it's through the HYH community or by some other avenue, the need for community is indispensible. My experience is that without it, you won't be able to overcome your problems with food.

You can learn more about how to become a part of the HYH community at www.healyourhungerbook.com

---

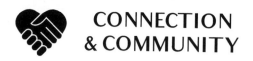
CONNECTION
& COMMUNITY

CENTEREDNESS

 CLEAN EATING

 COMMUNICATION

 CONSCIOUSNESS

 CAUSES

COURAGE

chapter 6

CENTERED*ness*

Finding a way to get centered amid the chaos and stress of everyday living is a vital element in overcoming emotional eating. In fact, it's vital to overcoming *all* addictions.

The biggest cause of emotional eating is stress, and the biggest cause of stress is a lack of self-care. How can lack of self-care be the culprit? What about all the burdens on our time and energy that always seem to befall us? Aren't they really the culprit? Well, in a word, no. Because life happens to all of us. It's how we handle life that determines our success or failure. And the best way to handle life's pressures is to be sure that we are rested, properly fed, emotionally supported, and spiritually nourished. And by *spiritual*, I don't necessarily mean religion. I mean a sense of well-being at your very core. If this has been a struggle or a block for you, stay with me.

> **LIFE HAPPENS TO ALL OF US. IT'S HOW WE *HANDLE* LIFE THAT DETERMINES OUR SUCCESS OR FAILURE.**

As a matter of fact, this whole book is about self-care. That's what stopping the destructive cycle of emotional eating really entails: caring for yourself so you don't end up overcommitted, stressed, resentful, and discouraged to the point of believing that food is your answer. The answer truly does lie within you and in how you live your life.

One of the first things Roy taught me is to start my day by getting centered and spiritually connected. He helped me adopt a personalized self-care plan that I practice to this day, every day. This is a way for me to get still and quiet and to tap into my higher self or spiritual source, if you will, so that I can have the resources I need to deal with and negotiate the stressors of life.

So often, people focus on the physical aspects of self-care, such as diet and exercise, but neglect the emotional and the spiritual. And yet, without addressing our deepest needs, we won't be able to sustain any physical changes we make. Because, remember, emotional eaters use food for reasons far beyond physical nourishment. We use it to treat our erratic emotions, stress, and frustrations. So we need to find a better treatment than overeating.

Unfortunately, we emotional eaters are notorious for neglecting our most basic physical self-care needs. We skip meals, stay up too late, and don't drink enough water. On top of that, we bottle up our emotions. We don't talk about what's on our mind, and we try to do everything ourselves, not asking help from anyone. No wonder that by the end of every day, we're comforting ourselves with food again!

WHY WE STRUGGLE WITH SELF-CARE

Why is it so hard for people like us to take proper care of ourselves? Simple: we don't feel that we deserve good treatment. We can treat everyone around us like royalty, but when it comes to ourselves, we settle for scraps. We don't take the time to treat ourselves with care, because we don't feel as though we matter enough.

We also may have learned poor self-care from those who raised us. Maybe they didn't care for themselves, or maybe they treated us in a way that sapped our self-esteem and left us believing that we don't deserve to be treated well.

That's why the key to being able to sustain a healthier way of eating is to lessen those backlogged emotions, as well as the burden of stress those emotions put on you every day.

SELF-CARE IS NOT SELFISH!

If you're like a lot of emotional eaters, you may feel guilty at the mere thought of taking time for yourself. It might seem selfish to focus on *you* with time and care that you could spend helping someone else.

The truth is, it's actually selfish *not* to take time for you. Why? Because when you go, go, go and do, do, do, you wear yourself down to the point that you can't be much help to yourself or anyone else. You wind up tired, overwhelmed, resentful, run down, and sick. And how can you really serve others in this state? You may go through the motions, pushing yourself to do just a little more each day, but you certainly don't feel happy. And when you aren't happy—or, even worse, when you're *un*happy and depressed—that doesn't serve anyone.

The reality is, it's a disservice just to give and never take time for you. When you take care of yourself, you have more energy for others. So you could say that self-care is really selfless!

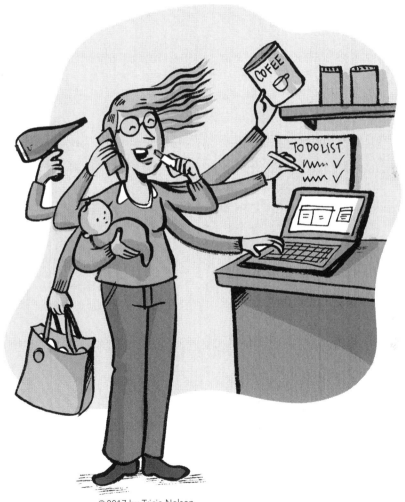

©2017 by Tricia Nelson

One small warning: even if I can convince you that self-care is not selfish, this doesn't mean that everyone in your life will be equally convinced. In fact, your family and coworkers—the people you spend the most time with every day—may not be so supportive of your new positive habits. No matter how much they love you or how great they think you are, remember, they have probably bene-fited in some ways from your *not* taking care of yourself and taking care of them instead! After all, emotional eaters are pros at taking on too much, saying "yes" to projects they don't have time for, and trying to be all things to all people.

So if you begin making changes that include saying no because you're trying to take better care of yourself, expect some pushback. You will feel torn between pleasing those who disapprove, and pleasing yourself and your body. At the beginning, your desire to please others will be stronger than your desire to please yourself After all, this is a strange new concept—you've never put you first. But if you persist and do what you know you need to do for yourself, and if you're willing to let some feathers get ruffled in the process, you'll eventually get used to your new self-care plan—and so will they.

For instance, after several months of meditating, the children of our client, Kim, noticed when Kim didn't meditate. She would be stressed and quick to anger. When that happened, they would say, "Mom, maybe you should go meditate!"

When you stay committed to your new habits, your loved ones start to notice the benefits *they* derive from *your* self-care. You are happier, nicer to be around. And things that used to upset you just roll off your back. Before you know it, your friends and family will be glad to support you in caring for yourself.

Oh, and by the way, eventually, Kim's kids wanted to learn how to meditate.

INTRODUCING YOURSELF TO SELF-CARE

The only way to get good at proper self-care is to *practice* proper self-care. Look at your calendar and see how full it is. Check out your to-do list and see how long it is. Is there anything scheduled that includes relaxing, being quiet, having time to just chill? Is there anything on your list that you can delegate to some-one else?

Self-care doesn't happen all at once. It's cumulative. And it starts with one step, one small act of self-acknowledgment and care. When you do that one thing, you boost your sense of self-worth a little bit, so that the next self-caring thing doesn't feel so foreign to you. If you took a half hour out of your day to have a cup of tea and leaf through a magazine, maybe you could take a half hour tomorrow to take a walk. And once you're in a pattern of taking twenty minutes in the morning to meditate, maybe twenty minutes later in the day can at least become plausible. It's one baby step at a time, so that the next baby steps become easier. How do you eat an elephant? One bite at a time!

THE SIX SELF-CARE SUCCESS SECRETS

I must make self-care a priority so I can truly show up for my life and for others. Every day, I do many things that support me, starting with my physical health, such as eating three balanced meals, taking the right nutritional supplements, and getting proper rest. Beyond those things, I do six very specific things that create the foundation for emotional well-being. These six things are part of my daily self-care routine. They ground me and help me feel connected to myself and my spiritual source. Without these practices, I feel ungrounded, foggy, and insecure—just the kind of mind-set that leads to overeating.

The reason these practices are so powerful is because they create an inner environment of peace and calm, which is essential for establishing an outer environment of sanity around food. When we are peaceful and our emotions are generally stabilized, food doesn't call to us. When we have taken the time to get

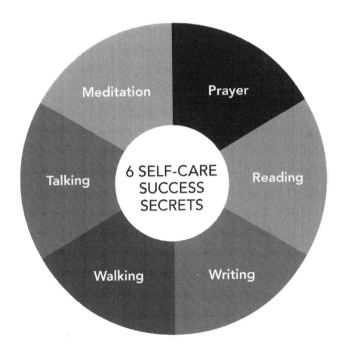

centered and to express our emotions in a responsible way, we are less likely to react to those emotions by overeating.

This comes with a caveat, however. On a subconscious level, we emotional eaters typically fear that if we actually do quiet down, the backlog of emotions we are accustomed to burying with food will come creeping back into our consciousness, making us even more uncomfortable. We have always overeaten to tamp these thoughts and feelings down, so doing something that might bring them up seems scary if not flat-out impossible. "If I quiet down, I'll be left with nothing but *me*." For most emotional eaters, that's a terrifying proposition.

Emotional eaters are busy people for this very reason. We run circles around other people, keeping a full schedule at all times. While it may seem as if we had no choice but to be busy and stressed, it's more likely that we choose this way of life because the busyness distracts us from our racing mind and destructive thoughts and obsessions.

But eventually, that busyness will take its toll—not only because the stress drives us to binge eat and gain weight, but also because no one can move at such a breakneck pace without eventually crashing and burning.

These six self-care practices are easy to do, cost nothing, and have only positive side effects. I have therefore affectionately named them "The 6 Self-Care Success Secrets."

SELF-CARE SUCCESS SECRET #1: MEDITATION

There are many positive ways to release anxiety, and in my experience, meditation is one of the most powerful.

Why do I attach such importance to meditation specifically? Because I've found that meditation has a wondrous effect on the mind, body, and spirit. Many people think meditation is some strange ethereal practice. The truth is, all kinds of people meditate every day. Presidents of companies, academics, Hollywood producers and actors, and prominent sports figures find time to meditate because it "ups their game" and allows them to get more out of life.

Meditation has many benefits, and not just for emotional eaters. Research published in a 2012 report in *Psychological Bulletin* titled "The Psychological Effects of Meditation: A Meta-Analysis" concluded that Transcendental Meditation practiced twice a day for twenty minutes reduces common anxiety, negative emotions, and neuroses, and improves learning and memory.

Research has also shown that meditation can help you achieve . . .

- improved brain function,
- better health,
- clearer focus,
- boosted creativity,
- more balanced moods,
- more happiness in life,
- stronger relationships, and
- inner peace.

There are many kinds of meditation, and even more books written about the various forms. Roy and I have been trained in multiple forms of meditation. We have meditated for decades using a silent mantra and love the simplicity of it. Many similar versions of this type of meditation are being taught nowadays.

Ultimately, whatever type of meditation you choose, in the words of my good friend and former client Vicki, it all boils down to the same thing: Sit down and shut up!

Many people who loathe the thought of sitting still will profess that they meditate when jogging, driving in their car, or brushing their teeth. Let me make an important distinction here between "mindfulness" and meditation. They aren't the same. Being mindful when washing the dishes, brushing your hair, or making dinner is a wonderful thing to strive for, and it certainly has its own mental and emotional benefits. Being mindful is about being in the present moment, bringing your mind back to here and now when it wanders away from what you are doing. This can decrease thoughts of worry and fear and increase feelings of joy and connection with a higher power and those around you. While mindfulness is certainly meditative, it isn't the same as the practice of meditation. Let's explore a little further how you can move past your resistance and begin to meditate.

THE ONLY WAY YOU CAN DO IT WRONG IS NOT TO DO IT.

Here are some of the most common objections to meditation that I hear. You may be entertaining one or two of them right now.

Meditation Objection #1: "I don't have time to meditate."

I often hear this particular objection from our clients because they have busy lives and many responsibilities. I like to quote the early-twentieth-century minister and spiritual leader Emmet Fox: "If you have no time for prayer and meditation, you will have lots of time for sickness and trouble."

The truth is, we always find time to do what we deem important. You always find time to do your job, right? That's because you know that it's pretty important to keep that paycheck coming in. And you seem to find time to eat, yes? That's because you place eating high on your priority list. And watching TV or going on Facebook somehow make it into your busy schedule, don't they?

> **IF YOU HAVE NO TIME FOR PRAYER AND MEDITATION, YOU WILL HAVE LOTS OF TIME FOR SICKNESS AND TROUBLE.**
>
> —EMMET FOX

So you see, it's a matter of priorities. You can make time for meditation when you realize how beneficial it is for your health, emotional balance, clarity, and freedom from overeating.

Since this is a book for emotional eaters, let me underscore the best possible reason for meditation: you will likely need less food, and feel more satisfied with your food, when you have a regular meditation practice. I would go as far as to predict that you'll consume two hundred fewer calories at dinnertime alone if you meditate after work and before entering the kitchen to cook dinner. What do you say to that?

Meditation Objection #2: "My mind won't slow down long enough to let me meditate."

News flash: everyone's mind races when they first begin to meditate! In fact, there are some days that my mind is still quite busy during my meditation. This is perfectly normal. The key is not to judge yourself because you're "doing it wrong."

You see, the last thing your ego wants is for you to settle down and subject your unruly mind to a practice of meditation. Your mind loves to hurl millions of thoughts and fears at you every moment of the day. This way, it can keep you worried and scared and under the illusion that your mind is actually running the show. There is no room for a spiritual connection when your mind is noisy and fancies itself to be "in charge."

Allow yourself to go through the uncomfortable stage of learning something as new and strange as sitting still. Let the thoughts pass through your mind, and don't worry about any individual one. Think of it as similar to watching leaves float downstream. Let them pass without focusing on any single one and without trying to determine how many leaves there may be. It has been said that having thoughts during meditation is actually your body's way of releasing tension and stress—like dreaming during sleep. So relax and let the thoughts come and go— and keep meditating. The only way you can do it wrong is not to do it.

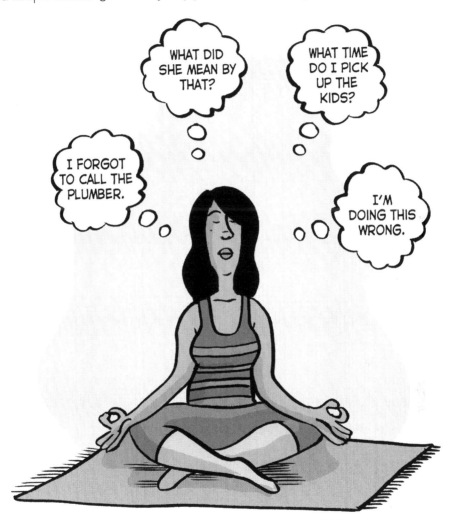

THE BEGINNER'S MEDITATION

© 2017 by Tricia Nelson

Meditation Objection #3: "I can't sit still long enough."

If sitting still and being quiet is new for you, you can work your way into it by starting slowly and briefly and gradually adding more minutes as you feel comfortable. Start by sitting quietly five minutes a day for a few days or even a week. These five minutes of quiet will make a big improvement. Then increase the time to ten minutes, and bump it up again until eventually you're doing it for twenty minutes. And by the way, when I say "sitting still," I don't mean you have to be in the lotus position. You can simply sit in a chair with your feet on the floor, or even sit up in bed with your back against the headboard. But be sure to sit (if you're physically able) instead of lying down—you'll stay awake more easily, and the benefit will be much more powerful.

The bottom line is, stop judging yourself as not being able to "do it right," and just start doing it. Five minutes of meditation beats no meditation at all. And if you stay consistent with it, you'll be able to sit for twenty minutes in no time.

Roy showed me how to meditate in 1988, and I've been meditating ever since. Meditation is probably the single most beneficial self-care habit I practice every day. It has transformed my health, my relationship with food, and my life. To help you get started with meditation, I want to offer you a recording of Roy walking you through a simple *Heal Your Hunger* meditation—the same way he taught me so many years ago—so you can experience how easy meditation can be.

Access your bonus recording on how to meditate at www.healyourhungerbook.com.

One more thing: I use a cool app that helps me time my meditation with various sounds such as chimes and gongs. So if, as you start on this new discipline, sitting in silence feels too difficult, the app also offers a wide variety of guided meditations and meditations with music, chanting, visualization, and other options. The app is called Insight Timer. It also lets you track the amount of time you spend in meditation, and even connects you with other meditators throughout the world. I highly recommend it.

SELF-CARE SUCCESS SECRET #2: PRAYER

Prayer is another amazing tool for creating calm in your life.

It is said "there are no atheists in foxholes," meaning that when push comes to shove and we find ourselves in a really tough or life-threatening situation, we resort to prayer.

However, when we're not in a "foxhole"—whether literally or metaphorically—some people pray and some people don't. And according to the research, people who pray have a leg up on the rest of the world when it comes to health and well-being.

Here are a couple of examples:

- According to Harold Koenig, MD, director of the Center for Spirituality, Theology and Health, out of over two thousand studies about prayer and health during the past decade, a majority show "a positive relationship between the spiritually uplifted mind and the body."

- A study conducted by the Harvard Medical School revealed that over 30 percent of Americans use prayer to help them heal physically, and in a survey of two thousand people who pray, a whopping 69 percent said prayer "greatly improved their health."

Yes, even in the scientific community, there is a growing consensus that prayer is powerful. Still, you may be wondering whether you need to be religious or believe in God to pray or to benefit from prayer. The good news is, you don't.

Prayer is actually nonsectarian. This may sound funny, but it isn't necessarily Christian or Jewish or Muslim or Buddhist. Indeed, it doesn't revolve around any particular doctrine at all. It's something you can do anywhere, at any time of the day or night. And it is a very personal experience—simply a statement of truth or of gratitude to some-thing that is greater than you.

REGARDLESS OF WHAT YOU BELIEVE OR DON'T BELIEVE, THE SIMPLE ACT OF PRAYER CAN HAVE A POWERFUL EFFECT.

The most universal prayer there is, is "Help me." Anyone can say "help me" without having yet figured out whether there is a God, what religion is right, whether God will actually help or even deems you worthy of helping.

What you may not realize when you cry out for help is that regardless of what you believe or don't believe, the simple act of prayer can have a powerful effect. It opens the channel of energy between you and a source of strength and power that can work wonders in your life.

If you're still uncomfortable with this, I understand. In my experience, all emotional eaters are to some degree leery about the whole topic of God and prayer. Some of us were hurt as children by people who were religious, or religion itself was used to hurt, scare, or manipulate us. Others have had bad things happen to them and may have decided that God wasn't there in their time of need. Perhaps you prayed for things, and nothing happened, and that reinforced your belief that God wasn't listening.

As a result, believing in God or depending on God may not seem like such a good thing. Truth is, all of us, including Jesus himself (Matthew 27:46), have had "God baggage." Fortunately, studies show that you don't have to believe in God to benefit from prayer.

So if you're a prayer novice, how can you incorporate prayer into your life? Just as with meditation, it's good to start simply. Try being grateful as a form of prayer. Think of things in your life that are good and that you can feel a sense of gratitude for. Gratitude itself is a powerful prayer that connects you with greater universal forces beyond your conscious mind.

You may want to begin redefining your ideas around God so that you can get benefit from opening a line of communication. To make it easier, remember that the word "God" is just a word used for convenience. But it doesn't matter what you call it: Spirit, Source, Loving Creator, Lord, Yahweh, Jesus Christ, Allah, Father, Mother, Father/Mother—honestly, it really doesn't matter. What matters is that you become open and willing to explore this relationship so that you can begin to take comfort from it.

As you might expect by now, I pray daily. But I'm not religious. I pray in my own way that feels sweet for me. I make a connection with God that comforts me and reminds me that God has my back. My goal is to keep this line of communication open as much and as often as I can.

It is the easiest, most accessible and readily available way I know to find and enjoy freedom from self-destructive thoughts and habits.

To access your prayer cheat sheet, as well as a chapter on prayer from Roy's book, *Love Notes from Hell*, go to www.healyourhungerbook.com.

SELF-CARE SUCCESS SECRET #3: WALKING

It may take thought, practice, and effort to meditate or pray. But there is another wonderful activity to help you get centered that is as simple as putting one foot in front of the other—literally.

Whenever you are stressed, upset, anxious, or depressed, going for a nice, easy walk—around the block, by the beach, in the woods, or wherever it's convenient—can help you settle down and feel more balanced. If you can walk in nature, even better. Studies have shown that going for a walk in a natural setting will bring you the most mental benefit. Regardless of where you choose to walk, you don't need to "power walk" or necessarily even break a sweat. It's more about the rhythm of walking, the fresh air, the conscious break from stressors such as phone calls (turn your cell phone off or leave it at home), emails, and responsibilities. This helps us reorganize our thoughts and our mood so that we come back reenergized and a little more balanced.

An article in *Monitor on Psychology*, a magazine published by the American Psychological Association, quotes James Blumenthal, a clinical psychologist at Duke University, as saying, "There's good epidemiological data to suggest that active people are less depressed than inactive people. And people who were active and stopped tend to be more depressed than those who maintain or initiate an exercise program."

I love to walk while saying my prayers. I call it my "walk/pray." It really centers me. I just walk around the block and talk out loud to God. (I put my earbuds in so people think I'm talking on the phone.) I say formal prayers that I've memorized, and I also just talk to God as if I were talking to my best friend. I tell him my fears, my thoughts, and whatever I need help with.

Whether you pray while you walk or not, walking is healing, and it's about as simple as you can imagine. It's great low-impact exercise, too. I like walking because it's gentle and not focused on effecting a change in my body (a perennial trap for the emotional eater). A couple of miles a day is my sweet spot. Not too much, but long enough for me to get the benefit on all levels. And now, using a telephone app or a Fitbit, I can even check how far I've walked. I love how technology has stepped in (so to speak) to make walking practically fun.

Because I feel so much better when I walk, I try to do it every day. It gives me energy, makes my bowels move more easily, increases my heart rate, improves my digestion, and definitely contributes to mental balance and an improved outlook on life. And when I combine it with my morning prayers, it's like putting on a coat of armor. I feel protected and calm, ready for a great day.

SELF-CARE SUCCESS SECRET #4: WRITING

Along with meditation, prayer, and walking, the practice of writing about our innermost thoughts and feelings is also wonderfully healing. Venting on paper is probably more powerful than the strongest verbal expression. Be it the anger, rage, sadness or even joy, writing down your feelings can help bring emotional balance very quickly. Important note: I do *not* recommend sending what you've written, especially if you wrote it in anger. Writing is so powerful that science and holistic medicine see it as a major route to emotional health and psychological well-being.

The holistic impact. As you translate your thoughts, fears, and emotions to the paper, your body cleanses itself of the pain, grief, and frustration attached to those emotions. In a study by J. W. Pennebaker and S. K. Beall in the 1986 *Journal of Abnormal Psychology*, interesting data emerged when groups of college students were asked to write about the most upsetting experience of their entire life. They wrote for only fifteen minutes a day, on four consecutive days. The researchers, Pennebaker and Beall, asked another group to write about only superficial issues such as their shoes or the condition of their room. The former group experienced a sharp decrease in visits to the college's health center, due to a much lower incidence of illness. Major reduction in the overall stress levels was also recorded. Pennebaker notes, "Writing gives structure and organization to feelings of stress and anxiety."

Facing your emotions. Your focus when writing makes a difference. Writing needs to be a no-holds-barred activity in which you simply write whatever flows into your mind. The best cleansing happens when you write without choosing your words or filtering your thoughts. A study in the 1999 *Journal of the American Medical Association* parallels Pennebaker and Beall's work. J. M. Smyth et al. had a group of seventy-one asthma or rheumatoid arthritis sufferers write about their stressful experiences, for three consecutive days. As expected, as many as seventy of the participants experienced improvement in their medical condition. Conversely, avoiding stressful emotions will push them back into the recesses of your subconscious. You can bet they will eventually resurface. (For more about this, see chapter 10.)

Another good reason to write? A recent study by Karina Davidson et al., in Lepore and Smyth's *The Writing Cure*, reported that expressive writing for as little as three to five minutes a day for four months actually lowered blood pressure and led to much better liver functioning.

Maybe you have been writing for years but still wind up overeating anyway. This is not because writing doesn't work—it does work, but typically not by itself. The difference is that when you combine the practice of writing with the practice of meditation, along with specific tools and ways of looking at things that I will share in this book, your writing will take on a deeper meaning and have greater power to change your emotional eating and your life.

Usually, people just write out the events of their day, pouring out their dreams or their unhappy feelings, and that's the end of it. This can be helpful, but there's a way for it to help even more.

When you write with the specific intention of searching for the pain, fear, and guilt behind those bad dreams or unhappy feelings, then writing can allow you to release these things. This is true especially when you also are seeking a deeper spiritual connection through meditation and prayer.

Writing is also tremendously helpful in dealing with feelings of rage and frustration. Usually, we take these feelings out on ourselves by bingeing. But writing out your volatile emotions can help take the heat out of them. Instead of raging at ourselves by bingeing or lashing out at some unsuspecting person (such as a loved one or a cashier at the store), go ahead and rage on paper. Write out all the negative, angry feelings you have. Write as much as you want, until the burn of what you are writing starts to cool down. You will eventually get tired of being angry and feel that the rage has deflated.

You may also see some things about yourself that were masked by the intensity of your feelings. You may see that the person you're angry at is *you (guilt)* or that underneath that anger is really *fear*. You may see that you're really just feeling hurt *(pain)* by a situation that occurred and that you felt powerless over. All these feelings that underlie the rage are "what's really going on," and writing can help access it. And once you have access to the truth of what you're feeling, you can begin to address it instead of stuffing it with food. You may even begin to see you have played a part in the situation.

Note: it's important that you keep your writing private and secure, where others cannot access it. Use a security code on your computer files or keep your journal in a hidden place. That way, you'll feel safer to let your true range of emotions out when you write.

Perhaps you're thinking, "That all sounds great, but I'd rather scale the side of a high-rise building than try to write." Well, you're not alone—but that doesn't let you off the hook!

It's important to know that you don't have to *like* writing to do it and benefit from it. Very few people, emotional eaters especially, *want* to sit down and write about their feelings. But as you write, the fury and jumble of your emotions will subside and you will become more centered. You will be more aware of what you're really feeling, you'll observe what moves you, and you'll become better able to make changes. And you'll start to be more accepting of who you really are: a child of God, simply doing your best.

YOU DON'T HAVE TO *LIKE* WRITING TO DO IT AND BENEFIT FROM IT.

You may hate to write, because you feel pressure to "sound good" or have everything spelled correctly. That's not what this kind of writing is about. This is personal writing—*for your eyes only.* You don't have to spell-check, use critical thinking, or even make sense when you write. And you can include as many curse words as you want. The key is to get the feelings out of you and onto the paper (or the computer.) Don't judge what you write. Just write!

SELF-CARE SUCCESS SECRET #5: READING

Reading can be very calming. But I'm talking specifically about inspirational literature—not gossip on the Internet or in *Us* magazine, and especially not the daily news online! Those sources have their place, but it's probably not when you need to quiet your mind.

I have a little cluster of books that I read a page or passages from daily. I actually read them out loud so I can better focus and integrate them into my consciousness. I also keep several spiritual books on my bedside table. I'll choose one before bed and read a few pages before turning out the light. When I fill my mind with positive, uplifting messages, I feel more connected to Spirit and more balanced emotionally.

Find some daily devotional readings, such as *The Daily Word* magazine, that offer positive words to help uplift you and inspire you throughout your day. Books with inspirational stories and positive messages will contribute to your sense of well-being and peace.

SELF-CARE SUCCESS SECRET #6: TALKING

Emotional eaters are good at keeping their thoughts and feelings to themselves. (Not their opinions, mind you—we have plenty of those!) But when it comes to how we really feel about things, we clam up. We judge ourselves and fear what others will think if we let the truth out, so we don't reveal much about who we really are. Obviously, this needs to change if we expect to stop overeating.

Talking about what's going on in your life clears the cobwebs out of your head. It eases your emotional burden and helps you get in touch with how you really feel about things. Here's a useful spin to the adage "garbage in, garbage out": When we accumulate emotional baggage and don't have an appropriate outlet, we become burdened and negative (garbage in), and food seems the only way to make ourselves feel good. But when instead we "put the garbage out" by writing and talking about it, we release that burden and quickly become positive again.

When clients come and talk to us about their day and they mention what inspiration they got from the writing they've done, they get further insight into who they are and what actions they want to take to improve their lives. The more they can share honestly, the more answers they receive. Not from *us* necessarily, but from that source of divine wisdom that lives inside them.

When you keep your thoughts to yourself, it's harder to access that wisdom. When you open up and let your thoughts flow and be heard, all kinds of answers are right there at the tip of your tongue.

Roy and I schedule time to talk together about our day, every single day. We have done this for decades, and we make a point never to miss a day. If we're in different parts of the world, no matter what time zone, we always manage to connect by phone, Skype, or FaceTime so we can talk through our day and give each other useful feedback when needed. We are committed to doing this, because we know how important it is to process our thoughts and feelings. As emotional eaters, we need to unburden ourselves of any negative residue that we may have picked up that day, either by ourselves or from situations we encountered. While this is obviously a good exercise for our marriage, we do it primarily because it enables us to keep our own emotional channels clear. This keeps us free from food obsession and best able to serve others.

Such is the power of talking as a self-care secret. If you decide to become a part of the *Heal Your Hunger* community you will have an opportunity to share your thoughts and feelings with other emotional eaters so that you can begin to heal.

You may decide that a therapist, close friend, or family member may be a better fit for you. Whatever forum you choose, just remember that isolation is the emotional eater's nemesis. You can't heal alone or in a vacuum, so the more pro-active you are about seeking support, the greater—and sooner—your success will be.

* * *

These are the six essential things you can do to help ease stress and tension throughout your day. There are many more out there, and different things may work for you.

Please note that I don't expect you to pick up all six success practices right out of the gate. That would be terrific, but unlikely and probably too overwhelming. Start by consciously trying to incorporate at least one or two of these techniques into your daily routine. The key is to make a consistent effort so it becomes a part of your day. If you're tempted to stop because you haven't lost fifty pounds after a whole week, I encourage you to keep at it. Besides, these aren't weight-loss secrets; they are success secrets, and they will have a positive effect on every aspect of your life, not just the weight. This is about a change in your lifestyle that will help you achieve and maintain emotional balance. The more centered you are, the less controlled you'll be by fear and stress, the two main drivers of emotional eating.

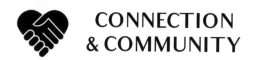

CONNECTION & COMMUNITY

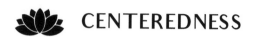

CENTEREDNESS

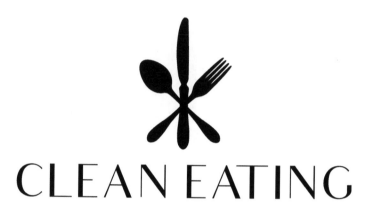

CLEAN EATING

COMMUNICATION

CONSCIOUSNESS

CAUSES

COURAGE

clean
EATING

Clean eating. The term implies that there's a way to eat that is clean, and a way to eat that is "unclean." So before suggesting what "clean eating" looks like, let's first explore its opposite.

Here's what "unclean eating" used to look like for me:

There was no beginning or end to my meals. I nibbled and snacked on whatever called to me (everything that was loaded with salt, fat, and carbs). Because I'm physically addicted to sugar, everything that had sugar in it captured my attention. It was hard to concentrate on the conversation I was having, because there was a bowl of candy on the table, and I really wanted some. If someone was serving pastries, I took one. I wasn't really satisfied with one, so I obsessed about having another, but I was worried about what others would think and whether they'd notice. I checked out how much others were eating, to gauge how much I could get away with eating. I tried to take another in a nonchalant way, as if it were no big deal, when in fact, it was all I could think about. I obsessed about how many calories I had eaten, and tried to limit my calories so I could "save" enough of them to eat what I really wanted (again, something loaded with sugar, carbs, salt, and fat). I ate a balanced meal when I was with my friends and family, but I stayed up later than I should watching TV or checking out Facebook. Then I'd begin to snack, which led to a seemingly endless binge. I woke up in the morning feeling bloated and sick, and disappointed that I hadn't gone straight to bed instead of eating. I watched the food channels and checked out recipes online because food was always on my mind, so I might as well get good at cooking it. I would often bake cookies, brownies, pastries, and cakes—not for the special occasions I pretended they were for, but because I wanted to eat them myself. I would offer kids close to me sweet things—going out for ice cream or buying a special kind of candy—as rewards, mostly because I was dying to stop and get something to eat.

As the binges progressed, I became less and less discerning about the quality of foods I ate. The local 7-Eleven would do just fine for quick and cheap junk food. And I was happy to use the drive-through window at a fast-food joint. (The more anonymous I could be, the better, lest someone I knew spot me buying massive amounts of food at odd hours of the day and night.) Sometimes, I would say something stupid to the person at the pickup window so they wouldn't think I was going to eat it all myself. So I'd make a comment like "My family can't wait for me to get home with this food," or "Marathon at work, and my officemates are starving." As if the kid at the window were remotely interested in what fictitious horde I was supposedly feeding!

Even when I tried to eat healthy, the only vegetables I desired were starchy ones, like potatoes, peas, or corn. I tried to control my portions of chips, cereal, and trail mix, but I would always end up eating far more than I had planned. A healthy lunch was usually a sandwich that included lettuce, pickle, and a tomato slice—basically the same as a salad, right? If I chose an actual salad (otherwise known as diet food), I added thick, creamy dressing, croutons, and cheese sprinkles whenever possible. I drank lots of soda—either the sugary kind because I preferred the taste, or Diet Coke for the hit of caffeine and the rationalization that I was being "good" since it was sugar free. At work, I would drink coffee to try to avoid snacking, but I'd add creamer and sweetener so it ended up being more of a milkshake than a cup of coffee.

I might go on a real health kick, eating a vegan, vegetarian or paleo-type diet. I'd buy all organic, maybe even try sprouting my own grains. I used only natural sweeteners and made raw meals and goodies containing raw nut butters, dates, cacao, and coconut. I pored over healthy cookbooks, looking for "legal" desserts that contained no grain, gluten, dairy, or sugar, and was quite proud of my culinary talents and my self-discipline.

But inevitably, my obsession with food and with my weight wore me down, and I gave up trying to be so "good." I would start allowing unhealthy foods into my diet, and before long I was bingeing on foods I had sworn never to eat (and that would have shocked my friends who considered me a healthy eater.) I felt embarrassed and afraid that I couldn't stop. So I would do a "cleanse" to get back on track.

Do these behaviors sound familiar? They're all various shades of *not eating clean.*

Add to these behaviors all the unwanted consequences such as feeling bloated, hungover, guilty, secretive, discouraged, obsessed, unable to concentrate, foggy brained, irritable, depressed, and hypocritical. And, yes, even suicidal.

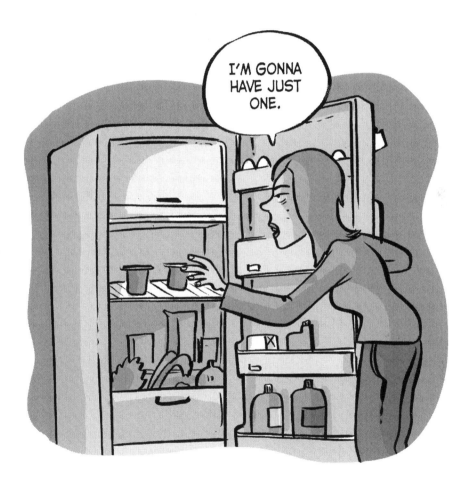

THE "JUST ONE" THEORY

© 2017 by Tricia Nelson

This is what sloppy, messy, or unclean eating looks and feels like. No matter what you call it, it's the pits. And yet, many people are living this way as a matter of course. It's a way of life, and over time they don't even question it. Sure, they try to control it, but if you're an emotional eater or food addict, trying to control it is like pushing back the tide. It's exhausting.

Of course, another word for "unclean" is "dirty." I don't call it "dirty eating," because that sounds too weird. But when you think about it, it's not far off the mark. After all, as a binger I certainly felt dirty, especially if my binge extended more than a day. I would let my personal hygiene go, including flossing and brushing my teeth and taking a shower. I got stains down the front of my shirt and on my pants from shoveling food in my mouth (and occasionally missing). I sweated as my body heated up from the intensity of all those carbs. I passed a lot of gas from eating foods that didn't agree with me, or eating something sugar free, which was sweetened with gas-producing sorbitol. So yes, you could definitely describe my eating as "dirty."

If your eating habits have been dictated by your emotions for years, eating properly may be a foreign concept. There's so much conflicting nutritional advice out there, you may be wondering what kinds of foods you should actually be eating, when you should be eating them, and what your relationship with food should really look like.

In this chapter, I'll outline some basic strategies that will help you make the kind of healthy food choices that will keep you thin, strong, and healthy—for life!

A PLAN DESIGNED WITH THE EMOTIONAL EATER IN MIND

Having been an emotional eater and having spent nearly thirty years in recovery and helping others heal, I am well acquainted with the traps and triggers that give emotional eaters the greatest trouble.

There's plenty of great advice covering what and how to eat from a nutritional perspective. Dieticians, fitness trainers, nutritionists, and doctors have oodles of viable, scientifically based plans designed to help people who are struggling with their weight.

The problem is, for most emotional eaters, those plans just don't work over the long term. Knowing the right foods and how much of them to eat isn't enough, because the emotional component of our eating defies all nutritional wisdom.

When we feel compelled to eat for emotional reasons, we couldn't care less about whether the stuff we're eating is "good for us." In fact, most of the time, we'd prefer that it *not* be!

Most emotional eaters would eat the right things, in the right amounts—if only we could. A lot of us have tried, and even succeeded at one time or another. But all that knowledge and sensibility goes out the window when emotions are churning and we feel the need to respond to those emotions with food. And no amount of nutritional know-how is going to break that cycle.

Most weight-loss programs are structured in a way that enables clients to answer their cravings with food. They provide a "cheat day" or suggest snacking on healthy foods when the cravings arise or the going gets tough. But what even the experts don't realize is that there is a way to *remove* the cravings for excess food or "cheat foods." When you heal the underlying causes of the emotional eating, those cravings can actually heal. And for an emotional eater, that is the only real, lasting solution.

> ## MOST EMOTIONAL EATERS WOULD EAT THE RIGHT THINGS, IN THE RIGHT AMOUNTS IF ONLY WE COULD.

As long as you stuff your emotions with food, even if that food is light and healthy and nutritious, it doesn't solve the real problem. In fact, it leaves the real problem unaddressed, thus requiring more food—or substitute fixes—to keep it buried.

Here's the caveat, though: to deal with the real causes, we need not to overeat. It seems like a paradox, doesn't it? You can't stop overeating unless you deal with the underlying causes, and to face these causes, you need to avoid overeating. Hmmm, sounds like the old chicken-or-the-egg riddle.

That is why I recommend a plan that provides the structure with which to overcome emotional eating. It's called Three-Meal Magic®.

THE MAGIC OF THREE MEALS A DAY
The foundation of the Three-Meal Magic® plan is eating breakfast, lunch, and dinner every day. No more, no less. No snacking in between, no satisfying urges when they arise. Now, if you're like a lot of people, you may be wondering why I recommend three meals a day when some experts recommend eating several smaller meals throughout the day.

The answer is that those five to six smaller meals work beautifully—if you're a "normal" eater. But if you're an emotional eater, the plan doesn't fit the problem.

The biggest thing emotional eaters need to learn isn't *what* to eat; it's *how* to eat what they know they should eat. It's the classic dilemma for the binge eater: "How can I do what I know I should do, and what my doctor, nutritionist, spouse, therapist, and friends suggest I do?"

The answer is simple: The only way we can eat the way we should is if we stop using food to deal with our emotions. And the only way to achieve this is to experience those emotions and face them, instead of stuffing them with food every time they pop up. This means that to *heal* your hunger, you're going to have to *feel* some hunger.

Eating several meals a day all day long won't allow that to happen. Because the whole point of near-constant eating is to keep hunger away. When we eat several smaller meals all day long, even if they're nutritionally balanced, our emotions are perpetually dulled to the point where we don't actually feel them. The result? We never have a reason to "go deeper" and look at the emotions under the surface that drive our cravings. It's not the hunger that emotional eaters are afraid to feel, but the emotions that the hunger reveals.

TO *HEAL* YOUR HUNGER, YOU'RE GOING TO HAVE TO *FEEL* SOME HUNGER.

If we are ever to heal, if we are ever to get past our emotions, we have to let ourselves experience hunger. But I'm talking about experiencing that hunger in a sane and healthy way, not by starving yourself, or even feeling uncomfortably hungry for an extended time.

That's the logic behind Three-Meal Magic®. The three meals are there to make sure you get the nutrition you need, on a predictable schedule. But since dealing with hunger is a huge challenge for emotional eaters, this plan is also designed to help you experience and get comfortable with the feeling of an empty stomach—and maybe even a few hunger pangs. Because, for emotional eaters, this is a positive (and essential) step toward healing.

That's the main difference between other experts' advice and mine. They don't always take into account the emotional reasons that motivate our eating habits; they focus more on what we're eating. So while they may provide us with good *nutritional* advice, that advice will only help us deal with *what* we eat, not with *why* we eat. So ultimately, that advice, as logical as it may be, can't translate into effective weight loss for people like us.

Three-Meal Magic®, on the other hand, does work. Here's how:

- It takes the guesswork out of meals and makes eating more structured.
- It arranges your day so you aren't either eating or thinking about food all the time.
- It eliminates a lot of the foods we tend to eat between meals, such as nuts, candy, chips, and chocolates.
- It gives your digestive system time to rest between meals.
- It shrinks your stomach since you're not stretching it with erratic binges, and a smaller stomach feels full on less food.
- It teaches you to feel and coexist with hunger and learn to distinguish between physical (real) and emotional hunger, and the difference between "hungry" and "full."
- It gets you to a point where you actually prefer the empty-stomach feeling of "hungry" over the stretched-out feeling of "full." (Trust me, it's possible!)
- It disciplines your mind, so you no longer need to give yourself everything you want, whenever you want it.
- It lets you enjoy your meals more. When you look forward to a meal and plan it, it tastes better.
- It keeps you aware of what you're eating and how much—something known as *conscious eating.*
- It helps you practice *finishing* your meal and moving on to another activity that has nothing to do with eating.
- It ends the deliberation about "whether I'm hungry and should eat."
- It helps you avoid "nighttime eating."
- It makes you more available to other people and projects since your mind can focus on something besides food.

THE THREE-MEAL MAGIC® PLAN

So just what *is* this magical plan? It's quite simple, really:

1. Eat breakfast, lunch, and dinner at roughly the same time every day.
2. Make your own meals whenever you can.

3. Make all three meals generally equal in size or calories so that your body becomes accustomed to that amount of food at each meal.

4. Allow thirty to sixty minutes for each meal, and take that time to enjoy it.

5. Wait four to five hours for the next meal, and don't eat at any time other than mealtime. In other words, NO SNACKING!

6. Stick to your schedule. Don't plan appointments when you normally have lunch, or decide to go to a movie when you usually eat dinner.

7. Get up early enough to sit down and eat breakfast before you start your day.

8. Make sure your meal is peaceful and quiet. Avoid distractions, such as people talking or coming and going, dogs barking, or children squabbling. Obviously, you can't control everything, but do what you can to create a calm, peaceful environment where you can enjoy your meal.

9. Try not to get up and down when you're eating. It's stressful and also bad for your digestion. Make sure you have your condiments, salt and pepper, water, and whatever else you need at the table, *before* you sit down to eat.

10. Don't answer the phone. Better yet, turn your phone off.

11. Eat consciously. Always eat sitting down and stationary—not in your car (unless you're parked), on the bus, on the subway, on the train (unless you have a seat and twenty to thirty minutes before your stop), and don't eat when you're walking. Don't watch TV (especially news) or read while eating. Or, if you need to read something, make it inspirational literature, not gossip magazines! Feed your soul while feeding your mind.

12. Inhale air, not your food! Sit up straight and breathe so your face isn't hovering over your plate. Put your fork down between bites and take a breath. This will slow you down and help you digest your food.

13. Don't drink a lot of water during your meal (a glass of room-temperature water is okay if you have challenges with digestion), and wait at least an hour before you begin to drink liquids. Water dilutes the digestive enzymes you need to digest your food.

WHEN THE GOING GETS HARD . . .

Three-Meal Magic® is easy: eat three meals a day, every day, at the same time, and nothing in between. But just because it's easy to grasp doesn't mean it's easy to stick to, especially in the beginning. This plan is about progress, not perfection. Learning to deal with your emotions and practicing effective self-care will certainly help you make that progress. When even that is not enough—

and believe me, those times will occur—here are some strategies to help you through the tough times.

If you're going to a party . . .

- The best recommendation is to call ahead to the hostess, chef, or party planner and find out what meal will be served, and at what time. That way, you know what you're in for and can plan accordingly. If you have special food needs, mention them to the chef or host, and see if they can accommodate your needs.

- If they're serving foods you would rather not eat or might be tempted to eat, you can always eat before the party. No one really cares whether you eat or not—especially these days, with all the various food sensitivities people have. You can just mention that you ate before you arrived. But if that's not possible or practical, skip the hors d'oeuvres and eat just dinner. If dinner will be served late, adjust your schedule by eating lunch a little later than normal so you're not famished by dinnertime.

- Concentrate on enjoying the *people* at the event instead of obsessing about the food.

- Remember, no one really cares whether you eat or drink.

- Three magic words that will get you out of a food jam: "No thank you." NOT "I'm on a diet," or "I don't eat that." Don't be righteous.

- Not everyone will be eating dessert. People who watch their weight don't eat dessert, and you don't have to.

If you're going to be away from home at mealtime . . .

- Plan ahead. (Failing to plan is planning to fail.)

- Always have a backup plan for traveling, for eating out, for emergencies. Don't be caught unprepared.

- Put care and effort into getting the food you need – try places like farmers' markets, natural grocers, and gourmet and specialty stores.

Wherever you are . . .

- Be willing to pay more for healthy, nutritious food. You're worth it.

- Drink water. (Dehydration makes you hungry).

STRATEGIES TO AVOID UNCONSCIOUS EATING

- Don't eat things in bags or boxes.

- Don't eat at your desk or while working.

- Put your food on a plate.

- What you eat on an airplane, in the air, counts. (I used to think it didn't!

- Don't shop for food when you're hungry.

WHEN FACED WITH A FOOD YOU KNOW YOU CAN'T HANDLE SAFELY . . .

Don't eat it. Whether it's chocolate toffees or barbecue potato chips or french fries or Girl Scout cookies, you can tell yourself you'll eat "just one." But seriously, when has that plan ever worked before? In my experience, "none is better than some." In other words, it's easier not to start than it is to stop.

WHEN YOU FEEL THE CRAVING TO OVEREAT . . .

Before you head for the fridge, take a moment to remind yourself that cravings don't "just happen" (even though it feels as if they do).

Cravings are of two kinds. They are physical, when you have sugar or carbs in your system, triggering an addictive reaction, or they are emotional—responses to thoughts and feelings that you want to hide from. And it's important to note that unless you've been sugar free for some time, your cravings will likely be both physical and emotional.

CRAVINGS DON'T JUST HAPPEN.

Since emotional eaters, by definition, are eating habitually to avoid uncomfortable emotions, it's likely that most of your cravings are reactions to your emotions. Which is nice to know, but what do you do about it?

When you feel cravings for certain foods that aren't healthy for you, try to remember the PEP Formula for digging a little deeper into the cause. Ask yourself whether you are craving food as a *painkiller* for emotional pain that you feel, as an escape from fears, or as *punishment* for some form of guilt?

You may be reading this and think, "That's silly. I'm not plagued with any guilt; I really just crave some chocolate!"

I understand. I've been there. I know from experience that at first, this idea of emotions lurking beneath your cravings will seem foreign and even a little strange.

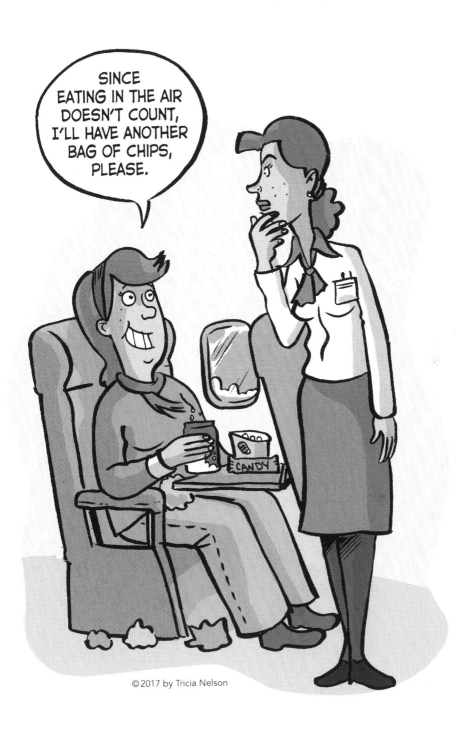

©2017 by Tricia Nelson

But humor me here. Remember, *cravings don't just happen*. You have thoughts that trigger emotions, and those emotions make you react from an unconscious belief that food will dull that emotion. That's a craving—in this case, an unconscious desire to *avoid experiencing* an emotion.

Most of the time, those thoughts and emotions are rooted in pain, fear, or guilt. Your ex showed up at the party with a new girlfriend, and suddenly you feel so much hurt that you reach for dessert. You must make a phone call to close a sale, and you're so anxious that you dig into a carton of ice cream to steady your nerves.

If you pause for a moment the next time you have a craving, chances are, you'll begin to notice what's *really* bothering you.

WHEN YOUR FAMILY OR FRIENDS DON'T SUPPORT YOUR NEW, HEALTHY FOOD CHOICES . . .

It's a letdown when the people we expect to be our biggest supporters try to undermine our progress. It's also very common.

In a survey of 1,226 respondents, conducted by eDiets.com, over 51 percent reported that friends regularly tempted them with off-limits foods when they were dieting. And 62 percent said it was far easier to stick to a weight-loss plan when they kept it a secret.

There's a good, if somewhat twisted, reason for this. When one person in a relationship starts to lose weight, it disrupts the status quo. Especially when the issue of food and weight is relevant to that relationship.

There are subtle psychological dynamics involved when one person is always struggling and the other is the cheerleader, the "strong one." When that dynamic shifts, it threatens the status quo and the role of the "strong one." Your friends and family members aren't used to your growing strength and self-confidence, and may feel uncomfortable.

Also, their own weight issues may be harder to deny now that the focus isn't on you and your weight issues. They may compare themselves to you and feel like a failure, and this could trigger their subconscious desire to sabotage your progress.

The best thing to do, for both you and the relationship, is to be quiet about your new path. If this is truly a lifestyle change, then you need to be committed to it no matter what anyone else says or does. And that includes making hard choices. If you don't want to eat at a restaurant or party that isn't safe for you, it's okay to say no or to bring your own food.

And it's also okay to distance yourself from people who are negative. Your own well-being has to come first. If you stay on course, others will eventually become reconciled to your changes and may even join you.

WHEN YOU FEEL SO HUNGRY YOU JUST CAN'T DEAL WITH IT . . .

This new way of eating takes time to adjust to, and there may be some days when you just can't stick to it. If you feel as if you'll die if you don't eat something, then eat something like an apple, or drink a cup of almond milk. Choose something that has a beginning and an end, as opposed to, say, a handful of nuts, which is apt to turn into four handfuls!

Then, to avoid the same situation tomorrow, try to examine how you can structure your day differently so that you don't get so hungry. Look at how much time you have between meals. If it's more than six hours, you're probably not going to make it without needing a snack. So see what you can do to have a more balanced meal schedule.

> **WHEN I INTENTIONALLY STAYED AWAY FROM FOODS CONTAINING SUGAR, I FOUND IT EASIER NOT TO OVEREAT.**

Also, you may simply not be eating enough during each meal. By trial and error, determine how much food or how many calories you can eat in a day without gaining weight, and then divide that amount by three. Or, if thinking in terms of calories is a trigger for you, try just eating amounts that are consistent in size at each meal. Trying to eat that same amount at each meal ensures that you don't get too hungry between meals.

It's important to get clear about safe foods and slippery foods. Safe foods are those that you can take or leave. They don't call to you or trigger fantasies about eating them. The ones we obsess about are our slippery foods. Obviously, many foods cause mayhem for emotional eaters. Especially seductive are the ooey, gooey, chewy ones. You can easily identify them. Slippery foods, however, are in more of a gray area. They may even be healthy and legitimate for most people. But for you, they spell *danger*, because once you start eating them, you have a hard time stopping. Or they preoccupy your mind for a good part of the day as you anticipate eating them, even though you likely have more important things you could be doing with your time. For instance, fruit might be safe, while nuts might be slippery. I have found over the years that when there is something I like "too much"—meaning I can't wait to eat it and it's all I think about—it might be a slippery food for me, even if it's healthy. So you have to get honest about your "safe" and "slippery" foods and honor that. Or perhaps I should say, *surrender* to that, because for emotional eaters, giving up foods that we're attached to is more a surrender than a choice.

This is also when being part of a community can save the day. Being able to jump onto a private group online and let others know your struggle, and receive immediate support and encouragement can make the difference between a binge and a "clean eating" day.

IF YOU FALL OFF THE WAGON . . .

First of all—and this is important—never beat up on yourself if you overeat. Overeaters overeat. But berating yourself for it will only set you up for more guilt, which leads to more bingeing. Remember the "P" for "punishment"? We overeat to punish ourselves for the guilt we feel.

The best thing to do if you fall down is to talk about it with someone who will understand the importance of what you are feeling. Then look for which emotions were bubbling up inside you and may have caused you to reach for the food. Use the overeating "incident" as a teaching tool, an opportunity to learn about yourself and what makes you tick. Since cravings never just happen, what feelings were you resisting or denying? What was your anxiety level? What thoughts were racing through your mind that you wanted a break from (escape) by eating?

Incorporating this new way of eating into your life won't always be a smooth transition. You're human and you're learning, so you're going to hit some bumps. But as you use the tools provided in this book and as you learn to rely more on the Seven C's than on food to deal with your pain, fear, and guilt, Three-Meal Magic® will become a mainstay in your life.

WHAT ABOUT SUGAR AND FLOUR?

Many people ask me about cutting out flour, sugar, and many sugar derivatives.

When I was nineteen years old, my sister went to a treatment center for food addiction. My mom and dad and I attended daily classes and nightly meetings alongside my sister for a week of her stay there. They called it "Family Week." Well, that's the first time I learned about sugar: how addictive it is and how prevalent it is in so many of the everyday foods we eat—products such as cereal, condiments, soups, and even many "health foods." That was certainly an eye-opener for me. From that point on, I wasn't so cavalier about eating cereal, ketchup, or canned vegetables. I read the labels and looked for products that didn't contain added sugar.

That was one of the most important pieces of information I ever learned in my life, before or since. Not that it kept me from ever eating sugar again, but my consciousness was raised and I was much more careful about the foods I ate.

When I intentionally stayed away from foods containing sugar—not just the usual sugar-laden culprits, but also those with hidden sugars, such as corn syrup, dried cane syrup, cane syrup solids, molasses, and honey—I found it easier not to overeat. Many foods such as sauces at restaurants, chewing gum, and salad dressings have either sugar or hidden sugars added. I had a much easier time with food cravings when I avoided anything with these sugars in it. It became evident to me that there was a definite physical component to my cravings. Sugar is highly addictive. Indeed, studies have shown that it's as addictive as heroin, so when I ingested it in any form, I was setting my body up to crave more of the same. And as you know, trying to resist cravings, whether emotional or physical, is close to impossible.

Yes, even the FDA is getting clued in. According to the FDA website, "scientific data shows that it is difficult to meet nutrient needs while staying within calorie limits if you consume more than 10 percent of your total daily calories from added sugar, and this is consistent with the 2015-2020 Dietary Guidelines for Americans." Added sugar in any amount can be a trigger for emotional eaters who, like me, are addicted to sugar, but the point is that there's a growing awareness that eating sugar causes weight gain and contributes to many negative health issues.

It was the same deal for foods containing flour. At that treatment center, I also learned that processed flours convert quickly to sugar when ingested, so they set up the same physical cravings as sugar. I eventually found that this happens even with grains and starchy carbohydrates. While whole grains take longer than processed grains to break down into sugar, many emotional eaters such as I find that any kind of grain can still be addictive because it breaks down into sugar, thereby setting up a craving for more. This is one of the reasons why paleo and ketogenic diets are currently so popular among health experts. The lower one's sugar intake, the easier it is to heal from a variety of health issues, such as inflammation, autoimmune disorders, and hormone imbalances.

So the upshot is that when I avoid eating sugar or flour, I feel better. People tend to get scared by this notion, as if their sugar is going to be "taken away."

That's why I frame it in a different light—not as a gimmick, but because it's true. Not eating sugar is an act of self-care, not deprivation or punishment. Punishment, for me, is trying to eat small doses of sugar- or flour-rich foods (like "normal" people, which I am not). It's nearly impossible to eat these foods "in moderation," as doctors, nutritionists, and health coaches recommend. Great advice—if you're not a sugar addict or on the higher end of the emotional-eating spectrum. (Take the spectrum quiz provided at www.healyourhungerbook. com.) When it comes to sugar, I cannot moderate without a Herculean effort—an effort that ultimately, I can't sustain. But why would I even want to put myself through the needless torment?

NOT EATING SUGAR IS AN ACT OF SELF-CARE, NOT DEPRIVATION OR PUNISHMENT.

If you're having trouble with food cravings, consider that both sugar and flour are setting up a physical addiction that you're likely powerless to resist. Personally, all grains make me want more, so my eating is cleaner, and feels cleaner, when I leave them out. I'm not saying this is what you should do. I am saying you should consider this information in light of your own experience and overall self-care blueprint, which we'll work on later. Why put yourself at a disadvantage? Why set yourself up to fight and struggle with food?

Making this path as easy as possible is always the best bet, and accepting your own personal vulnerabilities around food is a form of surrender that will pay great dividends in peace and neutrality around food.

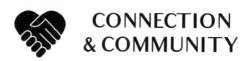 CONNECTION
& COMMUNITY

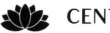 CENTEREDNESS

 CLEAN EATING

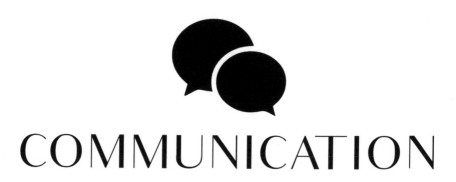

COMMUNICATION

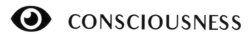 CONSCIOUSNESS

 CAUSES

 COURAGE

chapter 8

Communication

The number one common denominator among emotional eaters is our fear of honestly expressing our thoughts and feelings. We have plenty of *opinions*, and we may even feel free to voice those opinions frequently. But when it comes to expressing our *emotions*, many of us find ourselves at a loss for words.

In fact, the most common conversation for us is the one we're having *with ourselves* just after having an exchange with someone who was hurtful. We are busy thinking of all the things we "should have said." (Oh, yes, and don't we come up with some great zingers then!) We would have "put them in their place" had we just opened our mouths and said such-and-such to them!

But, of course, we didn't. Instead, we stood there smiling, acting as if we weren't hurt at all and everything were just hunky-dory.

Clear communication doesn't come easily to us. That's probably because a lot of us feel embarrassed by our emotions and judge them as being "silly," "not important," "a sign of weakness," or "whining."

Why? Well we may have grown up in a home where emotions weren't freely expressed, and if we expressed ours, we were teased, ridiculed, or even abused. In my husband's family, there were beatings to be had for making a wrong move or talking out of turn. In my home, I had a fear of being teased or scorned if my opinions differed from my family's, which made me ashamed of my true feelings and afraid to express them freely. Sarcasm (a form of veiled anger and aggression) was a common tone as well, which, at times, made it feel unsafe to be myself.

Emotional eaters typically avoid confrontation at all costs. It brings up too many feelings and situations that we can't easily control (such as other people's emotions). For that reason, we often feel that we need to agree with our families and friends and talk about the things they want to talk about. We assume that the more we go along with what others believe (all the while stifling our own true thoughts and feelings), the more accepted we will be. It's no wonder we wind up completely disconnected from who we are.

This is a common pattern for emotional eaters. Based on our conditioning in childhood, combined with an overall feeling of insecurity and fear, we do our best to avoid feeling vulnerable, instead keeping up a facade of unflappable self-confidence. As for our emotions, well, we use food to keep those nicely bottled up inside, of course.

But when we stuff our emotions with food, we lose touch with what our emotions actually are. This makes communicating them even harder. We are so disconnected from ourselves that we don't know *what* we feel, let alone how to express it.

The more disconnected from others and from ourselves we are, the more isolated we become. We withdraw inside ourselves, where we feel "safe." People close to us may try to draw us out, to get us to engage with them, but more often than not, they can't. Emotional eating keeps us uninterested in dealing emotionally with other people and with the world.

SAY IT OR STUFF IT

While our cocoon may seem safe and unthreatening, it's actually anything but. And to recover from emotional eating, we must come out of hiding. Being able to speak to a person (or people) we trust allows us finally to let out all the pain and self-judgments that we've been stuffing inside. And this relieves the pressure to numb our feelings with food. Being part of a community where this is encouraged and supported makes taking this crucial step easier.

Of course, learning to speak up doesn't happen overnight. It takes practice. But step by step, a little at a time, communicating honestly with others actually paves the pathway for dealing with our emotions, instead of eating over them.

In fact, self-expression and connection can actually *replace* food as a source of comfort when we feel bad. Once, early on when Roy was mentoring me, I had a compulsion to eat ice cream. It was so strong, I was sure I would have to give in. But I got in my car and drove thirty miles to meet with Roy instead. It was really

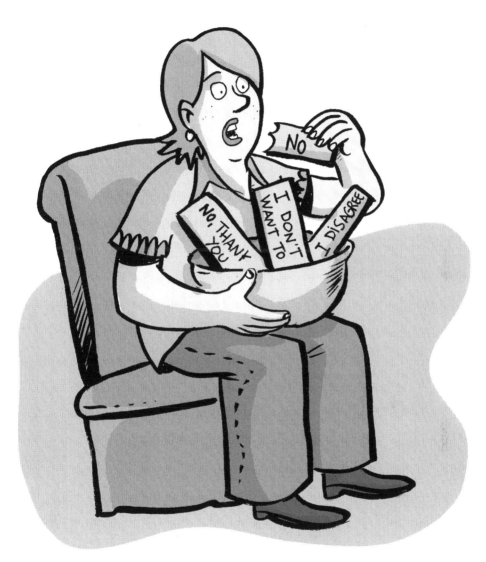

SAY IT OR STUFF IT

© 2017 by Tricia Nelson

late in the evening, but he was willing to see me. I told him about my compulsion and then started talking about the things that were bothering me. I talked and he listened, and then he shared experiences from his own life that helped me better understand what I was feeling. And the compulsion to eat ice cream subsided. Before long, I didn't even feel like eating. I was astounded. Expressing my jammed-up emotions—the same emotions that, when buried, were causing my craving for ice cream—helped me overcome my desire to overeat.

As we learn to identify and value our own opinions and desires, and to express them, we will see a ripple effect through every area of our lives. As an added benefit, the more accepting we are of ourselves, the easier it becomes to let others be whoever and however they choose to be.

To help you find your voice, here are my Ten Secrets to Expressing Yourself with Confidence. Remember them as you practice speaking up.

I. HOW YOU FEEL AND WHAT YOU NEED ARE JUST AS IMPORTANT AS THE FEELINGS AND NEEDS OF OTHERS.

"It's okay, it doesn't matter." If you're an emotional eater, you've probably used that phrase often when someone is rude, hurts your feelings, or ignores your needs. But is that really true? At the end of the day, when you sit down with a bag of popcorn and a gallon of ice cream, is it really true that those comments didn't matter?

IF YOU INTEND TO HEAL YOUR HUNGER, YOU CAN NO LONGER AFFORD TO DISMISS YOUR THOUGHTS AND FEELINGS AS UNIMPORTANT.

If you intend to heal your hunger, you can no longer afford to dismiss your thoughts and feelings as unimportant. You need to value them and see that you're just as good as other people—and that it's not appropriate to try to protect someone else's feelings at the cost of your own.

I'm not talking about being a rageaholic or being rude to others. I'm talking about speaking up without worrying about how other people will react. As emotional eaters, we tend to take care of other people's feelings. Maybe you think that if you speak up you'll make someone feel bad or uncomfortable.

Putting someone else's feelings ahead of your own in this way is "playing God." It's really none of your business how someone may react when you express yourself. Of course, there can be a situation when you might put yourself in physical danger by speaking your mind, in which case you might opt not to, but that would be a rare exception.

Hearing you speak up may actually help others. They may get a chance to see that they caused another person pain, and learn from it. But regardless of what your speaking up does for others, it's good for you. And that's the important thing.

2. YOU WILL NOT DIE FROM SAYING HOW YOU FEEL.

Right now you might feel, on some level, that honestly expressing your feelings to others will kill you, or that those feelings and opinions are so horrible they might kill someone else.

I'm here to tell you, that won't happen.

I'm not talking about being hurtful. When we're mean to other people, it hurts them and it hurts us. So we feel guilty. And to punish ourselves, we overeat.

But the simple act of saying how you feel will not kill you. I understand that at first, your mind may tell you it will. When that happens, just tell it, "Thank you for sharing"—and go ahead and speak your mind anyway!

Being afraid to speak up can go back to childhood. Maybe early on in life, you were punished or ridiculed for saying how you felt, and decided that it's not a safe thing to do. Well, this is adulthood, and it *is* safe most of the time.

Of course, there are times, say, in a work situation or in an emergency, when you may want to tell someone what they want to hear. Or you may just want to keep your mouth shut. I'm not talking about those situations.

I'm talking about the 99 percent of the time that it is okay—and important—to express yourself. It may take some practice, but it's only by practicing and speaking up that you learn that (a) you're not going to die, and (b) neither is anyone else. In fact, it's the best possible opportunity you have of truly living.

3. YOU WILL NOT DIE IF SOMEONE DISAGREES WITH YOUR OPINIONS AND DECISIONS.

Do you ever feel like you're nothing without the approval of others? It's a common feeling among emotional eaters, sometimes dating back to childhood. For example, if you're one of those people who was (or still is) terrified to do or say something that would disappoint your parents, your spouse, your kids, or your boss, you may bend over backward to avoid disappointing those people.

But you can live through other people's disappointments. You probably have already lived through disappointing your parents, since every child does at some point. You can live through disappointing your spouse, your kids, even your boss.

AT FIRST, PEOPLE WHO ARE USED TO THE OLD YOU MAY FEEL THREATENED BY THE NEW YOU.

If you're an overeater and you disregard yourself and who you are, the food will be staring right at you. It's always there to remind you whenever you're not living in tune and in alignment with yourself and who you are.

So just know that when you do what you feel is right, when you follow your heart, even if other people may disagree, it's okay. You won't die from their disagreement.

Even better, although it may be scary, when you do it you'll get stronger, and the fear that you're going to die if you do it will get weaker, making it easier to do next time.

4. WHEN YOU FOLLOW YOUR OWN HEART, OTHERS ADJUST.

At first, people who are used to the old you may feel threatened by the new you. Again, I'm not talking about being obnoxious or doing things that are hurtful to other people; I'm just talking about following your heart.

But when you do speak up, your relationships change. When people who are used to hearing you say, "Oh, it's fine, no problem," suddenly hear you start saying, "That's not okay with me," and speaking up with some self-confidence, they may get a little uncomfortable. Because suddenly, you're not going to be so agreeable—and they're not going to get their way as much.

So they're going to have to do some adjusting. They're going to have to work a little harder in their lives. And that's okay.

You don't owe *anyone* not being true to yourself. You have to put yourself and your well-being first. So even if the people in your life grumble a bit, *they'll get over it*. They just want to gripe a little to see if they can get you to give up your new course and go back to the way you were, which is more comfortable for them.

But if you stick with it, if you persist in doing what is right for you, they will eventually settle down and get used to your new ways. In fact, they will even respect you for them!

5. BY BEING TRUE TO YOURSELF, AND THRIVING BECAUSE OF IT, YOU WILL SET AN EXAMPLE THAT INSPIRES OTHERS TO BE TRUE TO THEMSELVES.

You don't know what a disservice you do when you don't follow your heart. When people around you, such as your kids, your spouse, and people at work, see you acting as if you were worthless, when they see you putting yourself down and acting from a place of low self-esteem, it hurts them. When people know how much potential you have and they witness you not living up to it, they feel pain.

But when you live up to your potential, when you step up and speak up and live with boldness, others will cheer you on. Think about when you've seen an inspirational movie such as *Rocky*, or read a story in which someone overcame a weaknesses or handicap and lived with boldness. You root for them and feel exhilarated, because watching these characters overcome their obstacles ignites the hope inside you that you, too, can overcome. It turns on a switch inside you that says, "Yes, I can do this!"

> **YOU DON'T KNOW WHAT A DISSERVICE YOU DO WHEN YOU DON'T FOLLOW YOUR HEART.**

So remember when you're stepping out and you're thriving, when you're living according to your dreams and aspirations, that divine spirit inside you is propelling you forward. When you listen to that spirit and you say "Yes!" others around you will also be changed.

There are will always be more barriers to overcome and more fears to walk through, so give other people the inspiration to face their challenges by seeing you doing it yourself. Your gift of changing is also a gift to others.

6. IT IS NO ONE'S RESPONSIBILITY TO READ YOUR MIND, SO SPEAK UP!

This is probably the biggest communication issue for emotional eaters. We're afraid to say how we feel, and we expect other people to read our minds. We manipulate and control and are "passive aggressive" instead of simply being direct and forthright about our needs. This causes stress, tension, and guilt—which results in overeating.

As emotional eaters, we don't tell people what we want. We just want them to know already! We want our partners to read our minds and do whatever it is that we want them to do. We want our parents to give us the love we think we should have, and love us in the way we think we should be loved. We have a whole agenda for everybody around us, but we never bother to express any of our feelings or needs to them.

> **YOU CAN'T BLAME OTHERS FOR NOT DOING IT YOUR WAY WHEN YOU'RE NOT EVEN WILLING TO TELL THEM WHAT YOUR WAY IS.**

The thing is, you can't blame others for not doing it your way when you're not even willing to tell them what your way is.

Of course, your telling them doesn't mean they're going to do it, but it feels a lot better to put it out there, and it's a whole lot easier for other people to help you and serve you if you at least express yourself.

When you have needs and desires, you have a responsibility to let others know what they are. That doesn't mean giving orders to other people (unless you're their boss), but if there's something you want, say it. Get in touch with what you want, and express it.

Change means letting go of game playing. Be straightforward and express yourself clearly, and see how much easier your life becomes.

7. RESENTMENTS ARISE FROM NOT SPEAKING UP AND BEING HEARD.

As we learned in chapter 10, resentments erode your soul and your health.

We emotional eaters try not to come across as resentful. We're all about pleasing people and being agreeable. But underneath, we seethe with anger, thinking, "I did all this for you and you haven't done anything for me." And this attitude ends up seeping out of us, often by our being short or snippy when we feel wronged.

We do a lot for other people, but not always because we really want to give. Often, it's about what we think we'll get in return. We want credit, accolades, recognition. And we rarely get it, which leaves us in a constant state of turmoil and dissatisfaction. Which leads to overeating.

The solution is simple. If you're giving to someone, there must be no strings attached, however subtle. You can't come back later and say, "After all I've done for you . . . ," and expect something in return. If you ever catch yourself saying or even thinking, "After all I've done . . . ," stop right there and think about what's happening. Chances are, you have unspoken expectations of the other person because of something you did for them. You were giving with the hope of receiving. You were giving *conditionally*.

LET'S FACE IT, WHEN WE'RE SELF-OBSESSED WE'RE NOT MUCH FUN TO BE AROUND.

You might also encounter feelings of resentment when you feel hurt and don't speak up about it. If you have a problem with someone, discuss it with that person. Don't blame them or sulk inwardly or talk behind their back. Just take responsibility for the feelings you are having.

Discuss your feelings with others until you feel resolved, and then MOVE ON.

8. PRACTICE LISTENING TO OTHERS.

It's easy to get so busy obsessing about your own feelings, what you want to say, and how others will perceive you that you completely overlook the ideas and feelings of others. "Did what I said sound okay?" "Did he just say that? What did he mean by that?" "Was that directed toward me?" "Do I look okay?" "Do I sound okay?" "I'm sure I sound like an idiot." We are so distracted with thoughts of ourselves, not to mention thoughts about food, that we can't be present with other people.

Let's face it, when we're self-obsessed we're not much fun to be around. So practice tuning in to other people and just listening to them. Trust that you will get what you need.

When you put aside thoughts about yourself and truly listen to other people, you'll find that they begin truly listening to you. When you show up for others, others will show up for you.

9. "SAY WHAT YOU MEAN, AND MEAN WHAT YOU SAY, BUT DON'T SAY IT MEAN."

When you're not used to speaking up, it can be hard to express yourself in a gentle way. That's because when there's so much pent-up resentment and hurt feelings, it's easy to come off as harsh or aggressive when you finally do speak up. With emotional eaters, it's often "feast or famine"—we don't speak up for years, and then when we finally do, we're like a fire hose!

With practice, you will get used to saying your piece and letting that be it. Right now, it's important to do everything you can not to say things in a mean or offensive way, because then you'll feel guilty—and we know what the cure for that is likely to be.

Saying how you feel is not really a big deal if you do it in the moment. But if you don't say something in the moment and end up gnawing on it for hours after, deciding to say something later—sometimes *days* later—is too late. The moment is gone. It's just not appropriate to go up to someone and say, "You know that thing you said three days ago? Well, I feel like blah, blah, blah."

I'm not saying you can't reopen a conversation, because that may be a critical step in your growth and in your communication with that person. I'm just saying that when you chicken out of speaking up in the moment, then muster your forces and blast them later, it's inappropriate.

So try to address things on the spot and say them nicely. You'll feel much better all the way around.

10. AS YOU BEGIN TO SPEAK UP, GIVE YOURSELF PERMISSION TO BE AWKWARD.

When people who have spent their lives stuffing their feelings learn to speak up, it doesn't always come out gracefully. If that happens to you, if you feel awkward and weird, it's perfectly normal. But that doesn't mean you get to give up and say, "This doesn't work."

Learning to speak up for yourself is a transition that's going to take some time. Know that at first you may stumble over your words, or you may not get your point across. People might look at you as if to say, "Yeah, and your point is . . . ?" But don't let that scare you away. Just keep on!

Malcolm Gladwell, author of *The Tipping Point and Outliers*, said, "Practice isn't the thing you do once you're good. It's the thing you do that makes you good."

You owe it to yourself to get it out. You owe it to yourself to participate in life and to have real feelings and real conversations. You deserve to be a real person, not just an obliging automaton that says, "Yes, yes, it's okay, it's okay, no problem, I'm fine."

So let yourself stumble, but keep at it!

Also, just because others may not agree with what you say doesn't mean that your beliefs are wrong. Don't apologize for your opinion. Resist the temptation to preface what you're going to say with a self-belittling comment such as "This may be a stupid thing to say but . . ." If you believe it or feel it, it isn't stupid. It's just as valid as what anyone else has to say. So just say what you need and want to say.

You embark on a new relationship with yourself and others when you respond from what is in your heart rather than react to what you think is on others' minds. Self-esteem comes from taking risks and being YOU, not from the approval of others. You will be amazed at the new freedom you feel when you are true to yourself and no longer depend on the opinions of others. Your own approval will become enough, and when it is, you will realize your true worth.

Get your *10 Secrets to Expressing Yourself with Confidence* cheat sheet at www.healyourhungerbook.com

---

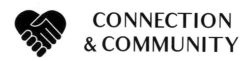 CONNECTION
& COMMUNITY

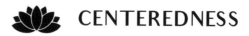 CENTEREDNESS

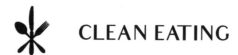 CLEAN EATING

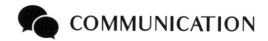 COMMUNICATION

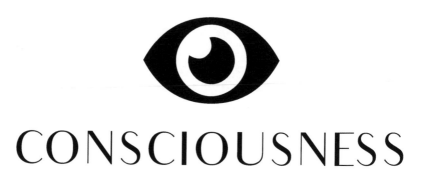

CONSCIOUSNESS

 CAUSES

 COURAGE

CONSCIOUS*ness*

The word "consciousness" gets thrown around a lot these days. It may seem a little "woo-woo" or New Agey since we often see it in the company of such terms as "chakras" and "spiritual energy." Not that there's anything wrong with such concepts, but consciousness is a lot more than just another New Age catchword.

The dictionary defines *consciousness* as "awareness of one's own existence, thoughts, feelings, and surroundings; full activity of the mind and senses, as in waking life; internal knowledge." This awareness of ourselves, the things we do, and how we relate to the world around us is an essential part of healing from emotional eating as well as other addictive behaviors.

The easiest way to understand the importance of consciousness for recovery from emotional eating is to look at what happens when it is missing from our lives. Lack of consciousness—lack of awareness of what we are feeling, thinking, and doing—is a huge contributor to emotional eating.

When we aren't conscious, we can easily consume the entire tub of popcorn at the movies, or a carton of ice cream in front of the TV, and not even notice how much we've eaten. As we get a little more aware of our bodies and our habits, it might occur to us that being stuffed is actually uncomfortable. But we still may not recognize that we feel bad about it.

In fact, you may have been in that very position when you picked up this book. You knew you had issues with food and needed to lose weight, but you didn't think too much about it until you read several of these chapters.

Maybe by now what I've been saying is starting to make sense to you. Maybe a few lightbulbs are coming on. Perhaps you've started reflecting on when you were a kid, and you begin to see how some of the habits you had then are contributing to your current problem. You may even have found yourself recently shutting the refrigerator door *without getting something to eat.*

What happened? Perhaps, after reading a few chapters, you put the book down and headed to the kitchen for a "snack," as you normally do. But this time when you opened the fridge, you suddenly heard this voice inside say, "Maybe I'm not really hungry; maybe I'm uncomfortable and looking to be comforted by a snack. I'm about to *eat emotionally.*" So you closed the door.

That is a change in consciousness.

You are now more aware of the connection between your feelings, your thoughts, and your actions. You know that your hunger goes deeper than the physical level. Voilà! Your consciousness has shifted.

In the past, you overate not only because you were unconscious, but also because it was a way to *stay unconscious.* Perhaps your reality growing up was so unbearable, and your feelings so intense, that you wanted to check out. (Remember "escape" in the PEP formula.) You thought being numbed out was the best way to cope with life, so you kept yourself filled with food, or at least obsessed with food, for years. I did this for the first two decades of my life. That's why, at the beginning of my path, I was unconscious of what I was doing to myself. I thought I "just liked food," until my sister came home one day and announced that she "ate over her emotions" and was trying to do something about it.

After that, I began to awaken to what I was doing, how I was eating, and the idea that it might not be normal or good for me. I was no longer okay with it. Over the next several years, it became increasingly uncomfortable, and I knew I must find a way to stop.

In fact, after beginning my recovery path, I fully awoke to the truth of what I had been doing to myself, and the terrible abuse I had put myself through. Not just with violent food binges but also with the compromises I made in relationships, the circumstances I chose for myself at work and in my living environment, and the decisions I made through my lack of self-esteem. I wouldn't treat my worst enemy as shabbily as I treated myself!

A DARK CONSCIOUSNESS

Sometimes, issues with consciousness go beyond simple numbness. We can enter a place in our consciousness that is so dark, we are aware that we're hurting ourselves or behaving in a destructive way, but we don't care enough to stop. For a food addict, that place can be so negative that we don't even *want* to stop.

This is a common state for people who suffer from all kinds of addictions, not just to food. We may be in such a dark place that we're actually conscious of punishing ourselves, of hurting ourselves, of making ourselves suffer, and we keep right on going anyway.

At that point, we are overeating for the very *purpose* of punishing ourselves ("punishment" in the PEP formula.)

Why would we do that? We will explore the reasons in the chapter on causes, but one major reason is that this is simply the inevitable progression of addiction.

Our emotional eating starts, in part, because we want to erase our consciousness. Our fear of *feeling feelings* is so powerful that we want to dull our sensitivity to all the things in life that make us feel things we might not want to feel or are too afraid to feel. At this point, overeating is a self-protective measure.

When that happens, food can actually save our lives. It can shield us from experiencing feelings that might otherwise be too much for us at the time and might finally cause us to snap. (Think mental illness and even violence—toward others and ourselves.)

The problem is that this self-protective distancing launches us on a vicious cycle. The more unconscious we become, the easier it is to numb our pain with food and other addictions. And the more we numb ourselves, the more out of touch we become. It can reach the point where we become so disconnected from everyone and everything around us that we completely lose our sense of who we are and what we're about. All we see is darkness. This may be the point at which we even consider suicide.

So what started as a means of protecting ourselves and our life ends up making us want to hurt ourselves and take our life. That is the powerfully destructive nature of addiction—and why choosing to stay unconscious can be a perilous decision.

If this is ringing a bell for you, I want you to know that *there is hope.* No matter how dark your consciousness has become, there is a way out.

The good news is that inside each of us, there's a place that refuses to fall *completely* asleep. You can look at it as a "spark of divinity," or a piece of the universal consciousness, or the Divine Mind, Holy Spirit, or inspiration. Whatever you like to call it, that "still, small voice within" may speak to us only in a faint whisper, but it is inside us, telling us what is true and guiding our way. It is our divine GPS.

> **WHEN WE LEARN TO LISTEN TO THE SMALL VOICE, IT GETS LOUDER. WHEN WE FOLLOW IT, OUR CONSCIOUSNESS GROWS, AND WE HEAL.**

We just need to wake up and pay attention.

When we learn to listen to this small voice, it gets louder. When we follow it, our consciousness grows, and we heal.

In fact, awakening your consciousness is necessary in healing from any addiction. You can't heal while living a life of darkness, self-neglect, and spiritual estrangement, but once you are on this path, you won't want to.

UNIVERSAL CONSCIOUSNESS

One of my favorite quotes is, "We're not human beings having a spiritual experience; we're spiritual beings having a human experience."

Another equally important part of becoming conscious is opening yourself up to the idea that you are not just an isolated being, living separately and distinctly from everybody else. In their book *Connected*, Christakis and Fowler write, "Our unavoidable embeddedness in social networks means that events occurring in other people—whether we know them or not—can ripple through the network and affect us."

Becoming conscious means seeing yourself not only as a human being, but as much more. You are a spiritual being who is part of a universal whole. And this means you must recognize that every thought and action that you put out affects the energy in the world.

I realize I'm sounding "woo-woo" again. But the idea isn't really so out there. When you're happy and healthy, that positive state affects everyone you come in contact with. Have you ever smiled at a stranger and had that stranger smile back at you? Remember how warm that quick, simple connection felt inside? Well, we all have within us the power to touch other people, which in turn touches us. Conversely, when your energy is dark, negative, and unhappy, it doesn't affect just you. It affects everyone you meet. Suffice it to say that we are much more powerful than we know, and our existence on this planet is much more important than we realize.

Being conscious also means awakening to the idea that a power greater than us is at work in our lives, and that this power is 100 percent good. I'm talking about the power of love—love in the largest, most expansive sense of the word. Knowing that this kind of love is out there, and that it surrounds us at all times, means that we are more protected than we know, more abundant than we can fathom, more loved than we think possible, more intelligent than we can understand, and far more capable than we believe.

Of course, people don't usually come to this realization all at once, like the Buddha receiving enlightenment under the Bodhi tree. They may have a burst of such spiritual consciousness, referred to at times as a "spiritual awakening," a "bright light experience," or being "born again." These instances are wonderful and can shift a person's consciousness so dramatically that it alters their behavior in an instant. This was the case with my husband, Roy. He had such an experience and stopped drinking and overeating, not to mention several other negative habits, in the blink of an eye, after sincerely and humbly praying to a God he didn't think he believed in.

But this is not how most of us awaken. Usually, it's a little at a time, through circumstances we experience and information we receive. That's why reading a book like this is so good for you. You are seeking information that can help you "see" from a new perspective. You are quite literally awakening as you read!

When you concentrate on things that are inspiring and *true*, instead of on the voices of negativity that you hear inside your head and all around you, your consciousness grows and expands. Then that new level of consciousness lifts your thoughts and actions to a higher level than before. So the actions that mirror your old, lower consciousness—actions such as eating that entire jar of peanut butter—don't fit with your new level of consciousness anymore. So you no longer feel compelled to do them.

In fact, *you can't do it*. When your consciousness is filled with positivity, doing self-destructive things feels too uncomfortable and strange, so you don't.

But remember, consciousness can be reversed, as well. Once you begin dabbling in "stinking thinking," being critical of yourself and others, gossiping, turning down good opportunities because of fear, feasting on political catfights, reading uninspiring literature such as celebrity gossip magazines, then little by little (and usually before you realize it), your consciousness will veer into a dark, cynical realm—until once again you're craving something sweet and heading back into the ravages of food addiction.

So it's important to keep a vigilant watch on the state of your consciousness. You do this by watching your thoughts, your words, and your actions.

The good news is, there are many things you can do to raise your consciousness, to fan that spark of divinity into a flame. Here are a few:

- Read spiritual or metaphysical books, magazines, and articles online (one of the Six Self-Care Success Secrets).
- Refrain from gossiping and being critical of others.
- Write a gratitude list and reflect on the things you are grateful for every day.
- Tell others that you appreciate them, and tell them often.
- Think of others' needs, and be helpful (when you can, without overextending yourself).
- Take a break from watching the news.
- When you're angry at someone, think of the situation from their perspective so you can acquire some compassion for them.
- Watch out for thoughts of "me versus you" and "us versus them."
- Focus on the collective "we" and the ways we all are connected with one another.
- Accept that there is more than enough to go around—enough food, enough love, enough attention, enough sex, enough money, enough jobs, enough opportunity, enough of every good thing.

These are not new ideas. You can find them everywhere, including in the Bible. One of my favorite passages is Philippians 4:8, where Paul writes, "Finally, brothers, whatever is true, whatever is noble, whatever is right, whatever is pure, whatever is lovely, whatever is admirable—if anything is excellent or praiseworthy—think about such things."

Remember, when your consciousness is fired up and expanding, you're far less likely to do things that are harmful to yourself. Healing becomes natural and virtually second nature.

A HEALING CONSCIOUSNESS

Metaphysical teacher and author Emmet Fox said that the circumstances in our lives are the exact *mental equivalent* of what is in our consciousness. If we have money problems, it may be that we have a "poverty consciousness"—a mentality that assumes a reality of lack and financial struggle. The same goes for our food problem. Our circumstances around food and weight are the mental equivalent of our current consciousness. If we have not provided the mental equivalent for freedom from overeating and for feeling lighter and more beautiful, we won't have this experience.

Real weight loss will be virtually impossible if we do not build a new consciousness—one that can accommodate a thinner body. Remember the statistic: 98 percent of the time, people who lose weight via a diet put the weight back on. Scientists, psychologists, physicians, and the National Institutes of Health are trying to understand why that is. To us, though, it's not rocket science.

The mental and emotional equivalent of food obsession, body hatred, and violent food binges is anger, self-pity, victim thinking, resentment, a desperate desire to control our circumstances, and an incessant need to get validation from others.

When we live in a consciousness of negativity and fear (a dark consciousness), that becomes a magnet for hardship and trouble. We make life hard for ourselves, our self-pity grows, and we moan, "Why do things like this always happen to me?" never realizing that our mind-set, our state of consciousness, is the reason. When our channel is clogged with negative emotions, it's more difficult for Spirit to flow through us and relieve our burden. And so, as emotional eaters, we need more food. It's that simple.

But maybe you work hard to stay positive and always have a smile on your face, and yet you continue to struggle. So this line of reasoning may not seem to apply to you. Given your positive outlook, things should go well for you, but the problem may lie in the emotions you have buried under your happy-go-lucky nature. You work day and night to do good things and bring a smile to others' faces, but deep down, buried pain, fear, and guilt are weighing on you. This makes you tired, stressed, and resentful. After all, you're working really hard and no one seems to appreciate you. This is a typical scenario for emotional eaters (and a textbook prescription for overeating). So being positive isn't enough. You have to dig deeper into your consciousness and heal what stands in the way of you and the transformation you desire. This is where the SOURCE work in the next chapter can really help.

OUR BODY CONSCIOUSNESS

The great motivational speaker Jim Rohn once said, "If someone gives you a million dollars, you'd best become a millionaire, fast!" His point is that we must have the consciousness to be able to handle the circumstances we want in our lives. Perhaps you've heard about the statistics on people who win the lottery, and how quickly most of them squander their winnings. This is because they have not built a consciousness that can accommodate that kind of wealth. They don't have the consciousness of a millionaire.

So if your goal is to become a thin person, you'd better become a thin person in consciousness. Unfortunately, those who grow up with a weight problem typi-

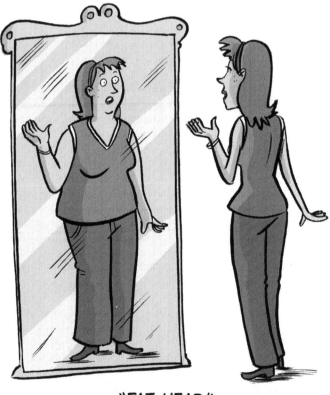

"FAT HEAD"
© 2017 by Tricia Nelson

cally have the consciousness of a fat person. I call this "fat head"—the inability to see ourselves realistically or judge our body size accurately. When we have a weight problem for many years, we unconsciously incorporate being fat as part of our identity. Sometimes, we don't even have to be fat to assume we are fat and build that into our consciousness. This was the case for me. When I look back at childhood photos, I find that sometimes I wasn't fat at all. I was normal size. But I always *felt* fat. And, of course, having the consciousness of being fat made it a self-fulfilling prophecy.

> **"FAT HEAD": THE INABILITY TO SEE OURSELVES REALISTICALLY OR JUDGE OUR BODY SIZE ACCURATELY.**

This is another reason why 98 percent of all diets fail. Because even though people may lose weight, they don't lose their "fat head" along with it. They still believe they are fat, still see fat when they look in the mirror, and still believe in their hearts that they will always be fat. Their identity as a fat person is burned into their consciousness, so even though they've lost weight, they are not at all comfortable or accustomed to having a thin body. It feels foreign to them. People tell them they look good, but they don't see it. Being normal size is disorienting. What's more, they no longer have the comfort that food and fat provided for them—the shield from others' attention, both sexual and otherwise, the buffer between themselves and their emotions, and the escape hatch from reality whenever things feel too real.

So when being in a body that feels foreign to them gets uncomfortable enough, emotional eaters have to return to the body they are used to, even if it's the body they spent so much time wishing they didn't have.

Emotional eaters end up overeating to reacquire the body that matches their consciousness of being fat—their "fat head."

So you can see how the consciousness that we cultivate by our thoughts, feelings, and actions can determine our relationship with food and weight. With a commitment to developing a new consciousness that supports our healing path, we can enjoy more health, happiness, and freedom from excess food and fat.

You can find a cheat sheet containing *10 Simple Strategies to Raise Your Consciousness* at www.healyourhungerbook.com

---

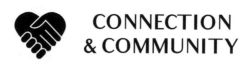 CONNECTION
& COMMUNITY

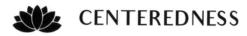 CENTEREDNESS

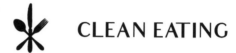 CLEAN EATING

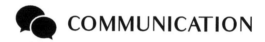 COMMUNICATION

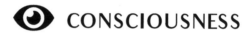 CONSCIOUSNESS

CAUSES

 COURAGE

chapter 10

Causes
(the SOURCE)

In chapter 3, we talked about the PEP formula that drives overeating: the need for a *painkiller*, *escape*, and *punishment*. We wouldn't need these if we didn't have inner pain, fear, and guilt that we use food to cover up. But what causes these difficult emotions? Do they just happen? Are we emotional eaters simply victims of these feelings that strike when they want to, whether we are prepared for them or not? It seems damned unfair that the emotional scales are tipped against us in this way.

Happily, that isn't the case—well, at least not completely. As we saw in chapter 4, part of the Anatomy of the Emotional Eater® is to be more sensitive and more fearful than the average person. But that doesn't consign us to an emotionally marginalized life.

From the beginning of this book, I've talked about disordered eating and issues with weight as being symptoms of the pain, fear, and guilt that emotional eaters are trying to bury. Well, guess what? The pain, fear, and guilt themselves are also symptoms.

To get relief from emotions that drive overeating, we need to dig even deeper to their SOURCE.

I have identified six of the most common reasons why emotional eaters end up with so much pain, guilt and fear. To heal these negative emotions and end emotional eating, we have to look at where they come from. Anytime you're having trouble or feeling out of control, take a close look at these six factors and you'll likely find the deeper causes, or SOURCE, of what's tripping you up.

(S) SPIRITUAL VOID

Most of the problems that I and our clients have encountered can be traced back to a spiritual disconnection. When we're not connected with a resource of inexhaustible strength, how can we ever get relief from our burdens?

When we have a spiritual void within us, we have a persistent feeling of emptiness. We feel weighted down by our problems and our emotions, and we don't feel much joy, if any at all. We go through the motions of living, but we don't feel any real connection to anything—to people, ourselves, or a higher power.

This spiritual void can afflict anyone, even people who are religious, including religious leaders. Sometimes, it just comes, but it is often triggered by a sudden tragic event or misfortune, such as a death, illness, or loss of a job. The most common reason for it, though, is that our ego has taken over and has begun to run the show. Character traits mentioned in Anatomy of the Emotional Eater®, such as being controlling and willful, snuff out any spiritual connection we may once have had. We will discuss ego in more detail later in this chapter (it's the "E" in SOURCE), but for now, we can think of "EGO" as the acronym for "easing God out." It is one of the most common ways that we have come to experience a spiritual void in our lives.

When we get into our ego and think we are in charge, we forget that there is a better, higher way. When we think that it all depends on us, we feel stressed and we take ourselves way too seriously. Our minds close and don't allow ideas or inspiration to flow in. Our work becomes hard, obstacles abound, and by day's end, we are exhausted by our attempt to control every last detail. We end up creating fear and guilt and pain, which we then use excess food to treat.

It's like a pond or lake that has an inlet and an outlet of fresh water. It will remain life sustaining with plants, fish, and an entire aquatic ecosystem. But when a lake has no flow, it becomes stagnant and unhealthy. When we are open to spiritual energy flowing in and out of us—you can even call it love, because that's what it really is—we, too, are like a living pond: energized, nourished, and refreshed. We have access to inspiration, guidance, and healing.

One of our clients, who had some bad experiences with religion as a child, was bitter about the whole idea of God. He figured he was better off depending on

himself than on some God that didn't really love him. This man also had problems with food, drugs, and his finances. After several months of working with
us, he finally decided to give God another try. But this time, he saw God as an
all-loving, all-knowing presence instead. The very next week, he was offered a
car, just at the time when he needed it. He attributed this wonderful gift to his
new attitude of openness, which helped him attract it.

If the word *God* makes you nervous, join the club! Most emotional eaters harbor
some mistrust in the idea of such a higher authority. This is often because that
higher authority came in the form of a bearded, judgmental man in the sky,
whom they learned about when growing up. But that's a scary thought for a sensitive, tender, guilt-prone little emotional eater such as we were back then (and
may still be!). This notion brought up so much fear, the only way to get relief
from the feeling that we were being judged by a taskmaster in the heavens was
to reject it altogether.

The good news is that spirituality has nothing to do with religion or even with
the word *God*. Spirituality is about the very things I'm talking about in this book:
connecting with your higher self, with love, with others, and with a deeper
source of strength and power that is infinitely greater than you. I often use the
word *God* because it's convenient, but my idea of what that word means has
changed dramatically since back when I was a kid sitting in a church pew. You
can use words such as *Universe, Source, Spirit, Great Spirit, Jesus Christ, Allah,
Father* (or *Mother*)—just about anything that feels comforting and true for you.
Roy calls it *Sweet Spirit*, which I love.

Try acknowledging this source during the day through prayer, writing, meditating, walking in nature, attending a spiritual service, or doing service for
others—anything that helps you reconnect with yourself and your spiritual
source. This will help you gain perspective and remember that the world will
operate just fine without you managing it.

Anytime you're having trouble with food or some other aspect of living, ask
yourself, *am I forgetting who I am?* That is, a spiritual being, loved and cared
for by my higher power. Or am I just operating by my own will? Am I moving
forward without any spiritual connection or consideration? Then pause and try
to reconnect.

My favorite thing to remember when things get tough is, "Don't tell God how
big your problems are. Instead, tell your problems how big your God is."

Roy and I have different prayers we like to say when we're down. But sometimes, all it takes is uttering the simplest prayer of all: "God, help me!" What you say isn't as important as the fact that you are taking time to acknowledge a source you can draw on that is greater and stronger than you. Try it. You'll be amazed.

DON'T TELL GOD HOW BIG YOUR PROBLEMS ARE. INSTEAD, TELL YOUR PROBLEMS HOW BIG YOUR GOD IS.

When you can remember that it doesn't all depend on you and that there is a spiritual source that can fill the empty place inside and make everything easier, you will think twice before turning to food to keep you going.

People usually expect God simply to heal their food cravings, but as I see it, turning to God helps us relax and make room for spiritual guidance, so that we no longer need the "support" of excess food. When we ask for help from Spirit, we can get out of our own way and see options in front of us that maybe we couldn't see—options that *don't* include overeating.

Many religious people who attend church or synagogue or some other place of worship weekly (or even daily) and who are obese might be a little miffed why, after all the praying, they haven't been healed. The reason is that it usually takes more than prayer alone. In the rest of this chapter, you will learn more about why spirituality alone won't heal emotional eating, and what actually will. But beginning to connect with Spirit will make exploration into the other aspects of SOURCE possible.

(O) OLD WOUNDS

Growing up, we likely experienced things that were traumatic, or at least very difficult to process. Usually, these things were so hard to process that we simply shielded ourselves from the pain as much as possible. While we may have used many different forms of "numbing," such as fantasy (daydreaming), masturbation, stealing, cutting, pills and alcohol, we usually turned first to food. We used overeating, bingeing and purging, or obsession with restricting our food intake as our first line of defense against the painful wounds of our childhood.

The problem with these various means of escape is that the pain didn't go anywhere. It was just temporarily masked, which means it stayed festering inside us.

Even if we weren't consciously aware of the pain as we got older, these wounds reared their ugly heads in the form of unhealthy decisions, knee-jerk reactions, and flawed character traits. Everywhere we went, we created chaos because of the wounds we suffered and the pain we buried early in our childhood.

For example, many emotional eaters experienced childhood sexual abuse. Michael D. Myers, MD, an obesity and eating-disorder specialist, estimates that 40 percent of his significantly obese patients have been exposed to or have experienced sexual abuse. Roy and I have seen an even higher percentage among our clients who struggle with food and weight, including those with eating disorders. Sexual abuse is a traumatic experience that triggers many conflicting emotions. Our clients who have experienced this trauma (including both Roy and me) usually responded to such a deep wound in one of two ways: either by becoming promiscuous or by shutting down and becoming asexual, or perhaps alternating between the two.

> Mary Anne Cohen, director of the New York Center for Eating Disorders, writes:
>
> Sexual abuse can have many different effects on the eating habits and body image of survivors. Sexual abuse violates the boundaries of the self so dramatically that inner sensations of hunger, fatigue, or sexuality become difficult to identify. People who have been sexually abused may turn to food to relieve a wide range of different states of tension that have nothing to do with hunger. It is their confusion and uncertainty about their inner perceptions that leads them to focus on the food.

The wounds of all forms of abuse, sexual or otherwise, that are buried yet remain very much operational in our lives, create what I like to call "hooks." We all have hooks in us that were left there by early childhood experiences. When we have these hooks, other people or outside stimuli can come along and grab on to one of them. Things someone does or says, or situations we encounter, can set us off in a heartbeat, making us feel angry, upset, needy, or even self-destructive.

WHEN YOU'RE HYSTERICAL, IT'S HISTORICAL.

In fact, few situations in our lives are really new. They are usually repeats of our past, based on our personal hooks. It has been aptly said, "When you're hysterical, it's historical."

Have you ever noticed that your boss reminds you of your father or your mother? The same feelings you had as a child growing up with an overbearing parent are all of a sudden being hooked by your boss, who acts in very much the same way. Or perhaps you have a friend who is overly critical and condescending toward you, much as one of your parents was. You feel as though you're experiencing déjà vu every time she throws a poison dart your way.

We all have had these experiences, and they aren't mere coincidence. We drew these scenarios into our lives based on our old wounds. We had hooks that someone was able to latch on to. This doesn't mean your boss isn't patronizing or that your friend isn't critical. It means that they are in your life because you have attracted them. The pain of your childhood is being brought to the fore because that wound has not yet healed. This seems unfair. You already had to experience it once, so why do you have to relive it in this new situation? But it's really a good thing. You are being given the opportunity to face and heal the wound for good, so that you no longer have to keep recreating situations that will "hook" it.

If you don't heal the wound, it will continue to fester inside you, causing symptoms that you will continue using food to escape from. Such symptoms could be sadness, loneliness, self-loathing, depression, anxiety and fear, or physical symptoms such as heart problems, hypertension, migraines, autoimmune disease, and even cancer.

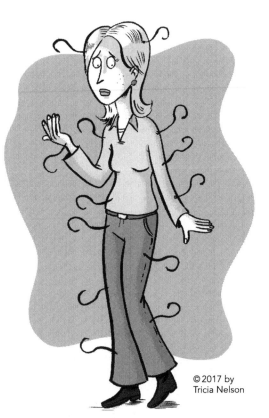

© 2017 by
Tricia Nelson

Our old wounds cause us to hurt not only ourselves but others as well. For example, we may sabotage new relationships by being mean or distant, because the pain of growing up in an abusive home made us afraid to trust.

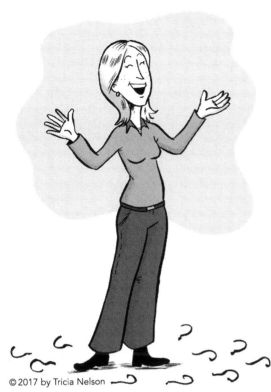
© 2017 by Tricia Nelson

The only way to stop recreating these experiences is to dissolve these hooks—to identify and dismantle them. Otherwise, we'll keep attracting people who hook us.

If you're feeling overwhelmed right now as you read this, it's probably because the last thing emotional eaters want to do is dredge up old wounds. After all, the whole reason we overeat is to cover up painful emotions. But don't worry, this doesn't all need to happen overnight. And you don't have to do it alone. In fact, you *can't* do it alone. The good news is, the specific tools and support this book provides, along with the safety of a community such as the *Heal Your Hunger* community, mean that it doesn't have to be overwhelming. And you won't need to approach it as yet another onerous task to do, either. Once you're on this path, the healing will unfold in a natural way.

The key is to find support in people who understand not only the problem of emotional eating but also that it is a symptom of deeper issues. It may be that a good therapist can provide the compassion and support you need to get started. We also offer "deep dive" programs that help you dig into this further so you can finally heal, once and for all.

After you have a safe support system of others, it's important to establish an environment of healing for yourself. In my experience, one of the most critical building blocks for emotional healing is self-care. When you have daily self-care disciplines that encourage peace, calm, and self-reflection, you will be better prepared for the inner work of healing. That's why it is vital that you work to incorporate the Six Self-Care Success Secrets into your daily routine. These practices will help you feel safe enough to slow down and let the old wounds surface so you can address them and finally heal.

The easiest way to start unraveling the pain of these old experiences is to use current situations as your guides. That cranky boss and the critical friend? They are now your newly appointed teachers! When you get hooked by their behavior, take an investigatory look within.

Write about what makes you feel angry or hurt. As you write, try to identify the familiar feelings that you have felt many times before. Try to recall what instances from childhood may have stirred the same feelings in you. Write about that experience. What happened? How did you feel? What were you thinking? What fears did you have? Let your pen flow on the paper, or your fingers click away on the keyboard, without any self-editing or qualifying. Don't hold back. Write until there's nothing more to say. Breathe. Let the tears flow. If you feel like it, curl up on your bed and have a good cry.

The key is to remember that whatever is showing up as a problem in your life today has emotional roots in the past. So it's an opportunity for healing if you will see it that way and take action, rather than considering yourself a victim. This is one of the great secrets to freedom from emotional eating.

(U) UNTRUE BELIEFS

We all operate under false assumptions—things we have decided about ourselves and others that simply are not true.

For instance, I believed at my core that I was stupid, bad, and ugly. (And most of our clients come to us believing the same things.)

Where do these beliefs come from? Well, usually from our childhood experiences. Our parents may have told us things in anger that were not true, but because we were young and couldn't discern the true from the false, we absorbed them into our psyche and believed them. Or perhaps we were raised by people who didn't have much self-esteem, and we modeled them.

My father placed a high premium on intellect. He and my sister went to Harvard. They were perceived as the "smart" ones in the family. The rest of us? Well, there were definitely some unspoken doubts! Because I wasn't quick on my feet like my father and sister, I was sure I was stupid. I couldn't argue my point of view with confidence, and I rarely aced a test, so in my mind, I lacked "smarts." And attending one of the top liberal arts colleges in the country didn't change that belief.

I also had convinced myself I was bad. I experienced childhood sexual abuse that left me with a ton of shame and a jumble of strong sexual feelings that I felt terribly guilty for having. As a result, I began to act out sexually at a fairly early age, and growing up in a religious home, I thought for sure I was permanently stained.

Another belief came up for me as well as for many of our clients who grew up with a weight problem: the conviction that I was ugly. Even clients who weren't overweight were haunted by this belief about themselves. It plagued us and caused us to shortchange ourselves at every turn in our lives. We settled for relationships or one-night stands with people we would never bring home to meet our mothers. We wasted years relentlessly obsessing about our looks, perhaps even paying thousands of dollars for cosmetic surgery.

It's hard for people who grow up fat to shake the belief that they're ugly. For me, it lasted long after I lost weight and my looks improved. It was especially hard to see myself as anything but overweight, even when my body was thin. In the previous chapter, I called this mind-set "fat head."

Yes, our untrue beliefs wreak havoc in our lives, and if we don't seek to change them, they will continue to cause problems.

I recently spoke with a woman who had many negative and detrimental beliefs about herself. And since they were *beliefs*, she was sure of them. No one could convince her otherwise. She couldn't even entertain the notion that they weren't *facts* about who she really was.

Early on in my own recovery, Roy would listen to me talk about something going on for me, and he would say: "You think you're bad, don't you?" And I would reply, "I *know* I'm bad." Being bad was not just a belief for me; it was a fact. I was so steeped in that belief, I couldn't view it as anything but true.

I can't say when that belief changed, only that it did change. First, it changed from being something I *knew* to be true, to something I *thought* about myself while knowing that it wasn't really true. And eventually, I came to know that just the opposite was true. Today I consider myself to be fundamentally good, intelligent, and beautiful. Sure, I have days when I am barraged by negative thoughts about myself. But I know they're not true. They are just a symptom of being overtired or having slacked on some of my self-care disciplines, so that I'm feeling disconnected from my higher power. Or perhaps I've been working too hard and feel distant from people who love me.

A good example of my evolving self-esteem is my process of writing this book. It has not been an easy task for me, mostly because of my lacking self-confidence. I wrote the first version of this book in 2008. After I printed out all the chapters and put it into a three-ring binder to begin editing it, I was so besieged by doubt, I literally put it on the shelf and didn't open it for five years! I had taken one peek at what I wrote, and thought, *this sucks!* And that was that.

I rewrote the book in 2013 and did basically the same thing with it. Then I got busy helping Roy write his book, which was a breeze—because it wasn't mine!

Finally, here I am in 2017, getting this baby ready for print, knowing that I can do this and do it well. To quote the Grateful Dead, what a long, strange trip it's been!

Understanding that your untrue beliefs are not actually true is the first step in changing them. But how do we do that? Experience has shown me that there is no bigger bully than self-doubt. So a feeling of safety is vital for us to begin unraveling unhealthy beliefs about ourselves. Unfortunately, we hold on to these beliefs as if they were our dearest friends rather than the bullies that they are. So to let them go, we must feel safe and confident that we can live without them, that we can venture into new territory with new beliefs that will expand our consciousness and our experience of life. There is no switch that can turn off these self-deprecating beliefs we have held for so long. They are deeply ingrained and take time to reverse.

THERE IS NO BIGGER BULLY THAN SELF-DOUBT.

As I learned, you can't do this alone. Having others around you who can hold a vision of what is actually true (that you are capable, good, and inherently beautiful) will make all the difference. This is why a community of supportive people is so vital. Let others be a mirror for you when your self-reflection is shattered.

Remember, once you commit to your healing path, you're on your way. But everyone's timeline for healing is different, so be patient with your progress. Also, should you want it and need it, *Heal Your Hunger* can provide a framework of support to help you progress on your path.

(R) RESENTMENTS

None of us can ever truly feel good about ourselves if we are holding anger and bitterness in our hearts. Nor can we overcome emotional eating. That's why the "R" in SOURCE stands for resentment. Clearing resentments from your heart is another important way to begin changing the untrue beliefs you have about yourself.

Feeling resentful is one of the most powerful, albeit subtle, drivers of overeating. Emotional eaters are always gnawing on all sorts of perceived insults and injuries, usually without being aware of it. We feel offended in seconds, often over practically nothing! It's part of our "victim thinking" that I talked about in the chapter on the Anatomy of the Emotional Eater®. Resentment causes a domino effect in our lives, with the reliable result of destructive eating.

Resentment is an emotional eater's greatest enabler, for several reasons:

1. We are prone to victim thinking.

2. We have strong emotions, so we're quick to feel injured, slighted, rejected, neglected.

3. We have unhealed wounds from our past that set us up to be hurt again (or to perceive that we're being hurt).

4. Because of our fragile ego, we tend to take things personally.

Emotional eaters are so adept at covering up their feelings in the attempt to be as pleasing as possible, the whole idea of being resentful may at first seem foreign. We tiptoe through our lives trying to be "nice," but all that "nice" has a dark side. We negate our actual feelings to such an extent that we have contorted ourselves into human pretzels, with a stockpile of bitterness.

The word "resent" comes from the Latin root *sentire* (to perceive or feel). So *re-sentire* is to "feel again."

Resentments are feelings of hurt and injustice that we repeatedly feel and rehash in our minds. They are injurious to the emotional eater because they fuel our disordered eating. How often have you binged "at" someone? Feeling hurt and self-pitying, you got out the food and drowned your pain. *But who were you really hurting?*

Even if you managed not to act out with food when in a state of resentment, think about the effect that feeling continually slighted has on your quality of life.

Living with a running list of offenses you perceive others to have caused you casts a pall of tension and sadness over your life. It's like walking around with a Santa Claus sack of bricks slung over your shoulder. And at some point, that sack becomes so heavy, you can't keep on moving. Depression seeps in, and you have trouble finding any joy at all in life.

Ultimately, the resentments we feel toward other people are really resentments we hold against ourselves, in disguise. While people have undoubtedly done us wrong, often we are mad at ourselves for allowing such shabby treatment in the first place—especially if we don't voice how we feel about it. Perhaps we had expectations of someone and they let us down. But if we hadn't held such expectations, we would not have put ourselves in a position to feel hurt. We may resent people who display traits that we ourselves have but that, blinded as we are by our righteousness, we cannot clearly see. We may find that we harbor resentments toward several people that are all of the same nature. Maybe they didn't love us or give us proper respect. In this case, when it seems to be a recurring scenario, it's likely a trait in ourselves that has caused the same kind of repeated resentment, or an old would that needs healing so we can begin to have a new perspective.

THE RESENTMENTS WE FEEL TOWARD OTHER PEOPLE ARE REALLY RESENTMENTS WE HOLD AGAINST OURSELVES, IN DISGUISE.

Roy often points out to clients: "You are the only person in your life who knows all the people you know. No one else knows the same combination of people, which means you are the common denominator in all the problems you have." Not an easy pill to swallow, but enlightening and freeing nonetheless! Because if we ourselves are the common denominator in all our problems, then we no longer have to see ourselves as powerless to change the situation. All we need do is look within and examine how we might change our perspective and our choices. Then we can stop being victimized.

You may suppose you have been so wronged that you have the "right" to resent a person. And the truth is, you do. You have the right to resent or hate anyone you like, or even a whole lot of people. But this mind-set won't heal your hunger. If anything, it will just make you hungrier! So long as you hold on to resentments, you are limiting your ability to feel joy and attract positive situations and people who treat you well. And you will certainly limit your ability to end emotional eating.

We aren't likely to be resentment free at all times. As long as we live and think, we will encounter situations that leave us feeling hurt, and we will be tempted to carry resentments. The key is to be mindful of your emotions and talk about them when you feel hurt. Using the Six Self-Care Success Secrets, you can process your feelings and then use prayer to help you let them go. Sometimes, that process will require speaking up and expressing yourself. For guidance on this, refer to the Ten Secrets to Expressing Yourself with Confidence.

The key is not to let wounds fester, but to address them so they don't drive you to food.

(C) COMPROMISE

Probably the most overlooked cause of emotional eating is the emotional eater's tendency to compromise—their values, their beliefs, and their inner guidance. There is no better shortcut to a marginalized life than to ignore your inspiration and listen to fear instead. Unfortunately, as emotional eaters, living this way has been the story of our life and one of the biggest causes of our troubles with food.

Remember, in the chapter Anatomy of the Emotional Eater®, when I mentioned the emotional eater's strong intuition, as well as the tendency to second-guess it? That's what I'm talking about here.

> **THERE IS NO BETTER SHORTCUT TO A MARGINALIZED LIFE THAN TO IGNORE YOUR INSPIRATION AND LISTEN TO FEAR INSTEAD.**

I believe that Spirit has a plan for us, and when we follow that plan, even when it's uncomfortable, our lives unfold in a harmonious, beautiful way. But when we ignore the signposts that are meant to direct and guide us, we run into trouble. This trouble creates disharmony and stress, hardship, and a sense of frustration, both creatively and emotionally. When we are out of alignment with ourselves and our divine purpose, we aren't in the flow, and our body, mind, and spirit will eventually break down.

Several years ago, a client came to us besieged by intense anxiety and depression. The best description for her state was that she was experiencing what is known in layman's terms as a "nervous breakdown." No doctors, medications, or therapists could help her.

She had always had a tumultuous marriage because, deep down, she never wanted to be married, and she was afraid to have children. And yet, she embarked on the life she thought she was "supposed" to have: marriage and children. Even though she had a career that she enjoyed, the stress of living a life she didn't really want weighed on her until she literally broke down.

WE SELL OUR SOULS OUT OF FEAR THAT WE WON'T GET WHAT WE THINK WE NEED.

When she began to tap into her inner guidance, her life began to change. She's still a mom and loves her kids, but she is no longer forcing herself to be married to a man she never wanted to be with. Even though he was good to her, she was still compromising her inner guidance by being with him, and it was making her sick.

When we aren't willing to listen to our inner guidance—otherwise known as following our heart—circumstances will arrange themselves to force us to listen. The good news is that you don't have to wait until you crash and burn. You can begin to pay attention and make new choices that set you free from your self-imposed bondage to a life that isn't truly you.

Many women make compromises when they feel societal pressure to get married and have children. Emotional eaters, especially, feel that their self-worth relies on it, that this is the only way they can feel "normal." They are far less discriminating when they feel desperate to be loved and accepted. Their need clouds their judgment when choosing a partner, and the ensuing stress and unhappiness can fuel their overeating for decades.

Marriage isn't easy and does require quite a lot of legitimate compromise. But when we compromise our values and our self-respect to have what we believe we should have, that's the wrong kind of compromise—the kind that causes emotional eating. To put it another way, we sell our souls out of fear that we won't get what we think we need.

We've all done it. We've all been afraid of what we would lose if we didn't compromise ourselves, and we rationalized the decision in a hundred different ways. But it's exactly those internal conversations that we have—when we feel bad for our decisions and keep trying to talk ourselves out of feeling bad—that tell us we are, in fact, selling out.

When we make compromises, we suffer. We feel bad about ourselves. We feel guilty, afraid, and worried. And before long, the stress of such emotions drives us to escape in food. If we binge enough, we will not only "forget" the compromises we made, but we will surely make more of them, because we are too numb to care.

This is the hidden danger of "selling out." People do it all the time. And it's always motivated by fear. We're afraid of our boss, so we stay late at work, week after week, even though it makes us late picking up our kids at school. We put up with crappy treatment from our boyfriend because we don't think we'll find anyone else if we break it off or even mention it. We stay in a job we hate, because we're afraid we won't find anything better. Our friend routinely blows off our lunch dates, but we go right on agreeing to get together, because she throws great parties and we want to be invited.

See the problem? In each scenario, we sacrifice our own self-respect, health, and sanity because of fear—fear of losing something or not getting something. We don't trust that if we put our self-respect, health, and sanity first, we'll be okay.

But the truth is, not only will we be okay, but we will be building a solid foundation of self-love and self-care that enables us to thrive. Because when we refuse to compromise ourselves, we build self-esteem and self-worth. This in turn gives us confidence to live boldly and to demand good treatment—from everyone. We won't settle for less.

And we won't need to punish ourselves with food.

Now, you may be wondering how to turn around the self-destructive compromises you've already made, without destroying your life in the process. You don't feel that you can just up and quit your job or get a divorce, so how can you make changes that enable you to feel better about yourself? The way to do this is to start recognizing the decisions you have made that perhaps were motivated by fear, and have compassion for yourself. Our fear-based decisions don't make us bad. We likely would have chosen differently if we'd had the self-esteem and confidence. From

> **WHEN WE REFUSE TO COMPROMISE OURSELVES, WE BUILD SELF-ESTEEM AND SELF-WORTH.**

here on, draw from your awakened consciousness and begin examining your motivations before making new decisions.

If you are in a marriage in which you have made many unhealthy compromises, try to see where you can begin making small self-caring changes. Can you ask for help with a chore that you normally do yourself but could really use a hand with? Are there responsibilities you can share more equitably? Maybe you could start by expressing your feelings about a situation you're not comfortable with—not expecting a certain outcome, but simply sharing some of your feelings about it.

You may want to see a therapist who can help you evaluate your choices, and support you in making new ones. If your spouse or significant other is open to seeing a counselor with you, this can help you begin to address the dynamics of the marriage in a safe way that isn't hurtful to either of you.

In other areas of your life, making changes as you go is the best bet. Challenge yourself each day to act with self-respect and self-care, even when you are afraid or feel resistance from others. Making compromises isn't necessarily a bad thing. It can be a healthy part of life and relationships—as long as you're careful not to agree to something that makes you feel bad about yourself or causes you to hurt yourself with food. No compromise is worth that.

(E) EGO

Ego is something that we emotional eaters often think we lack. Because we usually suffer from low self-esteem, we assume that we lack ego. But it's really just the opposite. People who have low self-esteem usually end up with *too much* ego—their inflated sense of self is compensation for their low self-esteem.

Ever heard someone speak of an "egomaniac with an inferiority complex"? Well, in my experience, *every* egomaniac has an inferiority complex. They may seem to think they are great, but if they were really convinced of this, they wouldn't need to work so hard to prove it to others and to themselves.

EVERY EGOMANIAC HAS AN INFERIORITY COMPLEX.

The truth is, the worse we feel about ourselves, the more egotistical we are. We name-drop so others think we're important, we drive fancy cars, and we wear expensive designer clothes and jewelry. We make sure to let people know how much we spent on our recent trip to Europe

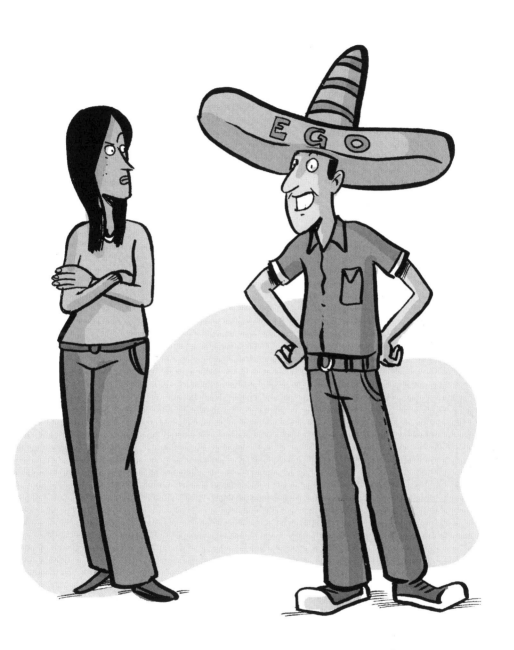

EGO IS NOT YOUR AMIGO

© 2017 by Tricia Nelson

or on a painting or a bottle of wine. We must constantly prove that we are special, influential, powerful, beautiful.

And yet, if we really felt this way, we would be content with the fact and go on about our business, instead of being so caught up with what other people think. If we felt secure in our own person, we wouldn't care what others think of us.

Our inflated egos routinely influence our actions, even if we don't act like big shots and are instead quiet and subdued. The way your own ego manifests will depend on your personality. Perhaps it will show itself as fierce competitiveness—the need to always be the best and get the most accolades, or the need to know interesting facts and trivia so you can impress people with your intellect. I'm not talking about the human quality of wanting to be well regarded and accomplished. I'm talking about an incessant *need* for these things—ego gone wild, so to speak.

Because emotional eaters are often so wounded and beaten down, we generally feel that we are less than others from the start. We compare ourselves relentlessly and usually fall short. Since it feels so bad to walk around feeling "less than," our ego is constantly looking for ways to steal a little boost from feeling superior to others.

So instead of having humility, we become self-aggrandizing (self-promotional). This way, we can pretend to ourselves and others that we really don't feel bad about ourselves, that we really are "all that and a bag of chips."

Unfortunately, this backfires on us, because while some people may believe our phony facade, many others can see through us.

This ego drama is a vicious cycle: we feel bad about ourselves, so we are boastful, defensive, and prideful. Then we feel guilt and self-loathing (whether consciously or not), which further lowers our self-esteem. Feeling even worse, we are even more apt to boast, defend, and try to prove our worth.

Of course, rejection from others because of these personality flaws drives us to seek solace in food.

The truth is that anytime we act from our ego mind instead of our God mind, we will display many unappealing character traits. See if any of these rings a bell:

- defensiveness (not being able to handle constructive criticism)
- taking it personally when someone disagrees with your ideas

- competitiveness
- comparing yourself to others
- seeking acceptance or approval from others
- feeling superior to certain people
- wanting credit for things you've done (and burning when you don't get it)
- envy of others' success
- feeling worse about yourself when others succeed
- subtly trying to pull people down with criticism or gossip
- being critical of others
- telling people what to do or how to do their job
- needing to be the best at something (or refusing to play at all)
- trying too hard to be funny
- jealousy
- impatience
- being a "know-it-all"
- blind, driving ambition

Again, these are human qualities that *everyone has.* It's just that emotional eaters, coming from a place of low self-esteem, tend to take them to the extreme. If you catch yourself indulging in some or many of these traits, go easy on yourself. Just recognizing them in yourself is huge progress, a giant step on your road to healing. Identifying aspects of your character that aren't pretty can be painful and may cause you to think you're a bad person. Nothing could be further from the truth.

The best illustration I've heard is Roy's combat analogy. (He's a former soldier.) Going into combat, the soldier wears a flak jacket, rifle, knife, helmet, and so on. It's a lot of gear to carry, but a soldier is happy to do so if it helps keep him or her safe. Then, once they're out of danger, the soldier sheds that gear as quickly as possible and chills out at base camp, wearing only fatigues.

When we feel as though we are in "hostile territory" because we're around critical people or just people who aren't emotionally sensitive like us, we feel as though we have to protect ourselves. The above character traits are just manifestations of fear, of not feeling safe to be who we are. So they don't make us bad; they just show what we think we need to survive.

When we feel safe, when we're around people who are loving and emotionally aware and who support our healing path (like those in the *Heal Your Hunger* Community), we can let down our guard and relax. No longer do we need our self-protective "gear" in the form of unappealing ego traits.

Another ego pitfall is that of being easily lured into doing more than our fair share when there are kudos or praise to be had from doing so. Because our self-esteem is so fragile, we tend to overcommit ourselves and do favors that we don't have the time or energy for. But with a little ego-stroking from others—"You're so good at this; can you help me?" or "You're always so dependable; I know I can count on you"—we're putty in their hands and will do almost anything, no matter the cost to us.

Weight loss is another area where ego afflicts emotional eaters. Because so many of us have spent time being miserably overweight and feeling inferior to our skinny friends, once we begin to lose weight it's not long before our ego kicks in and we imagine we're hot stuff. We go shopping for sexy, revealing clothes and love to put on our tight jeans to show off our awesome new body. Because we've rarely felt attractive, we become consumed with our new body and can't wait to be seen and admired. Unfortunately, we go overboard with self-obsession (and often sex obsession), and before long we feel empty and guilty—the perfect set-up for a binge!

The fact is, when we lose weight we are afraid. We feel exposed, unprepared for life without excess food, and so we scramble to make sense of the maelstrom of feelings that food is no longer keeping at bay. Our ego takes us on a wild ride that seems fun at first but ultimately sets us up for a nosedive.

If you remember Oprah's first experience with extreme weight loss in the 1980s, you may recall that during her show she rolled out eighty pounds of butter on a wagon, to provide a strong visual image of how much weight she actually lost. She was overconfident about her new body, which, unfortunately, bit her on the behind. She couldn't sustain the weight loss for very long. Let it serve as a cautionary tale.

I may appear to be saying that if you heal your hunger and lose the weight, you shouldn't be happy or proud about your accomplishment. Not at all. What I am saying is that one of the unsuspected reasons that 98 percent of all diets fail is that emotional eaters sabotage their weight loss because they fall victim to their runaway egos.

So be *grateful* for your weight loss but not *prideful* about it. And when you have feelings of superiority over people who haven't lost weight, pray to have that pride healed, because it's really just a sign of the insecurity that fueled your ego in the first place.

You may wonder whether it's even possible for people like us to develop a healthy ego. The answer is an unequivocal YES!

Steven Smith spent a decade exploring how great leaders use ego differently than everyone else. The result of his work is a book he cowrote with David Marcum, titled *Egonomics: What Makes Ego Our Greatest Asset (or Most Expensive Liability)*. In an interview with Smith, the author Guy Kawasaki asked him, "What is a 'healthy' ego?"

Smith replied, "Genuine confidence; confidence that doesn't have to exert itself to "prove" its confidence. Healthy ego keeps us from thinking too highly or too little of ourselves and reminds us how far we have come while at the same time helping us see how far short we still are of what we can be."

This is a beautiful description of the balance we all must seek as we negotiate life, business, and relationships. It may be a little easier for someone who isn't starting with a self-esteem deficit. Nevertheless, it is something we all can strive for. Based on a foundation of humility rather than ego, we can build a life that is healthy in all aspects of body, mind, and spirit.

As you can see, examining the SOURCE of your eating behaviors is not for the faint of heart. It's deep work and involves facing some not-so-attractive truths about yourself and your past. But as you do this, you will chip away the wall of emotions that has kept you trapped in the cycle of compulsion. You will free yourself from the burden of anger and shame that has fueled your heretofore mysterious cravings. There is a way for you to end emotional eating, and the SOURCE work holds the key.

If this work seems too daunting to do on your own, you're right, it probably is. That's why I developed an online course that is a companion to this book. It will take you by the hand and see you through these revelations and important changes. When you become part of the HYH community as part of the course, you will find the needed support to embrace this healing path. You have nothing to lose but a whole lot of baggage!

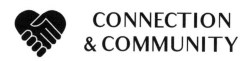 CONNECTION & COMMUNITY

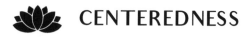 CENTEREDNESS

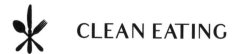 CLEAN EATING

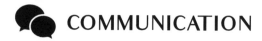 COMMUNICATION

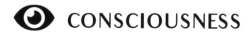 CONSCIOUSNESS

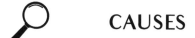 CAUSES

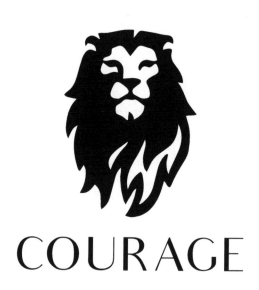

COURAGE

chapter 11

COURAGE

Courage is the last of the 7 C's. I saved it for last because it's the glue that makes all the other steps stick.

No matter how much sound information we take in regarding weight loss, emotional eating, food addiction, and eating disorders—including what's in this book—it will make no difference if we don't apply it. And the number one reason we don't apply it is lack of power, and its twin, fear.

The root cause of all our problems is fear. We don't do what we know we should, because we are afraid of walking through uncomfortable feelings to chart a new path.

Transforming your life takes courage, every step of the way.

But you don't need enormous reserves of courage. You just need enough to take the next step. And that's it!

You need enough courage to take an action that you don't want to take and that you don't necessarily even believe in. Just enough courage to say what you're afraid to say and to try something you've never tried before.

As we saw in Anatomy of the Emotional Eater®, emotional eaters tend to be riddled with fear. Healing requires that we walk through our fears, no matter how hard it may seem. I say "seem" because fear is a bully, and often whatever we're afraid will happen when we walk through our fears isn't even real. In fact, you can think of FEAR as an acronym for *false evidence appearing real.*

Having courage isn't an event. It's a recurring choice we make, which has a cumulative effect, like building a muscle. When you first exercise a muscle, it will feel difficult and might even hurt a bit. But if you continue to exercise that muscle, it gets easier.

It's the same way with courage. Courage is something we need to practice, but as we face our fears, that muscle of courage will grow stronger by the day. Of course, when we retreat into fear, the courage muscle begins to atrophy. So choose courage even when you don't think you can. By the way, this is a daily challenge, which all human beings must face.

It's important to note that courage isn't the same as willpower. I rarely can power my way through any situation, especially when I feel afraid. This is why I start my day by getting centered and connected with God. Being centered in Spirit gives me the ability to do things I'm afraid to do. While only I can have the courage to walk through my fears, that courage is fueled by my higher power. Therefore, I always say a quick prayer before doing something I'm afraid to do. It never fails to give me the "juice" I need.

Consider the words of the Serenity Prayer: *God grant me the serenity to accept the things I cannot change, the courage to change the things I can, and the wisdom to know the difference.*

Note that courage is the second thing we pray for. And not just courage, but specifically, *the courage to change the things I can.* This is because change takes courage—a lot of it. And since we probably don't have enough of it, it's not a bad idea to pray for more.

Consider all the moments on your *Heal Your Hunger* path when you will have the opportunity to practice courage. It takes courage . . .

- to feel uncomfortable emotions;
- to meditate when a voice in your head is screaming, "I can't possibly sit still;"
- to speak up and express your thoughts and feelings when you feel self-conscious;
- to examine your fears when someone else's behavior angers you;
- to reach out to others who understand your struggles, even though you feel embarrassed and awkward;

- to call ahead to the host of a party and see if they will be serving food that you can feel comfortable eating;
- to stop blaming others for your unhappiness and instead look inside to the root cause;
- to switch from sugar to stevia when you want to sweeten your tea;
- to let go of bread in your diet;
- to go to the farmers' market, buy vegetables, bring them home, chop them, and prepare a fresh homemade meal;
- to reach out for help when you'd rather figure it out on your own;
- to follow your heart and take a risk while your friends and family are cautioning you to make the safe choice;
- to change your holiday tradition and make it about the connection with family instead of baking all day as everyone expects you to;
- to leave the relationship and step out on faith that you can take care of yourself and forge a new path;
- to attend a social function when you feel shy and hate small talk;
- to write about your feelings and heartaches when all you want to do is dive into a pint of Ben & Jerry's;

REACH OUT TO OTHERS WHO UNDERSTAND YOUR STRUGGLES, EVEN THOUGH YOU FEEL EMBARRASSED AND AWKWARD.

- to pray when you're hurting, when you really want to slam doors instead;
- to refrain from gossiping about a coworker, because you know it's the right thing to do;
- to ask someone to take over a task or project, because your plate is already too full;
- to have compassion for someone who is behaving badly, and instead of judging, realize that they are probably acting from a place of pain;
- to call a friend who is struggling, even though you feel that you don't have the time;
- to get off the couch and go for a walk when you'd rather binge-watch your favorite TV show;

- to feel hunger pangs without reaching for food;

- to turn your problems over to a higher power instead of worrying about them all day;

- to say "I love you" to your spouse even when you're not feeling it;

- to turn off your phone when you get home from work, so you can focus on your kids and whatever kid things they want to tell you;

- to turn off your phone for a weekend so you can be more present and centered;

- to say no to another commitment because you're already stretched thin;

- to step down from a board or committee because you're tired and have already given plenty;

- to take actions that might cause people to judge you, because, from now on, what you think of you is more important than what *they* think of you.

Notice that very few of these acts of courage have anything to do with food. Yet they have everything to do with ending emotional eating. Every time you take contrary action by doing the opposite of what fear would have you do, you build courage, self-esteem, and faith. And little by little, you learn to depend on these inner resources instead of on food.

A willingness to be uncomfortable is one of the most valuable assets you can have as you set forth on your *Heal Your Hunger* path. Make a game of doing the uncomfortable things and facing your fears. Eleanor Roosevelt said "do one thing every day that scares you." If you're presented with something new and different, give it a try. Make a habit of it, so that stepping outside your comfort zone is no longer hard or scary, but simply a way to broaden your horizons and have new experiences.

And remember that you probably can't do any of this alone. Praying for courage and strength will help tremendously. Also, get support by being a part of the HYH community of emotional eaters who are forging their own new paths of courage. See how easy it can be when you link arms with others who are also walking through their fears. Know the exhilaration that comes from throwing off the chains of fear and saying YES to life and to you.

Only you can transform your world. But you don't have to do it alone. Let's do it together!

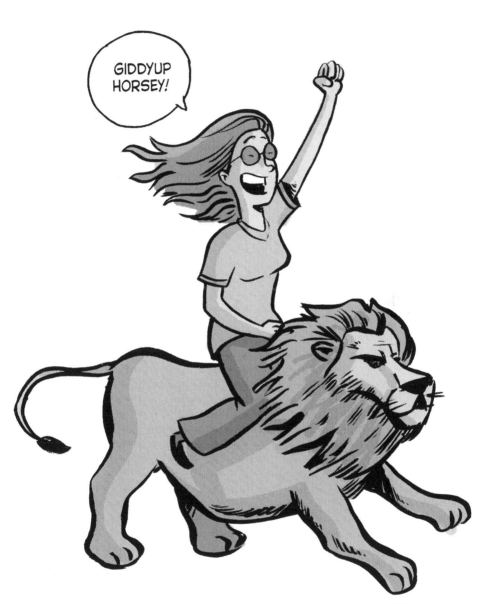

WHAT COURAGE FEELS LIKE

your HEAL YOUR HUNGER *blueprint*

Congrats! You've now learned the 7 Simple Steps to End Emotional Eating Now. These steps are your roadmap for how to heal your hunger and end emotional eating.

While "consuming" this information is the first step, you now must take action so you can make this new relationship with food a reality.

I have created an easy to follow blueprint below that helps you know what actions to take right now.

Also, should you desire help with following through on your HYH Blueprint, I have created a companion course that will take you by the hand and walk you through each of these seven steps so that you can break free from food cravings, get the support you need, and feel happier and lighter in every way, right now.

You can learn more about this course and access all the cheat sheets at www.healyourhungerbook.com.

YOUR HEAL YOUR HUNGER BLUEPRINT

Filling out this blueprint is for your benefit so you can begin to implement the changes suggested in this book. There is power in writing down the action steps you plan to take. You can alter your course at any time, but go ahead and get started now.

CONNECTION & COMMUNITY

Check off who you can connect with who will understand your struggles from personal experience and give you the support and encouragement you need.

☐ **Heal Your Hunger community**

☐ **Friends** (close friends, colleagues)

☐ **Family** (parents, siblings, spouse)

CENTEREDNESS

Meditation: Refer to page 80. Check off what kind of meditation you will try.

☐ Traditional (breath work, body scanning, letting go of thoughts)

☐ Guided (visualization, going on a path)

☐ Mantra based

☐ Chanting

☐ Heart Rhythm Meditation (heart beat rhythm, emotional)

☐ Online & Apps (headspace.com, insighttimer.com)

Timing: When will you meditate? (For best results develop a regular routine)

☐ Morning (before children wake up, after breakfast, on the way to work)

☐ Afternoon (during lunch, mid afternoon)

☐ Evening (before dinner, after dinner)

Prayer: Refer to page 84. Make a list of people and things you want to pray for each morning (For ideas about how to pray refer to the materials provided in the bonus link.)

☐ Loved ones (children, partner, family, friends)

☐ Lifestyle (sane eating, new job, healthy body, safety)

☐ Spiritual (connection with Spirit, divine guidance and wisdom)

☐ Mental & emotional (compassion, tolerance, forgiveness, positive outlook)

☐ Global (environment, people in need, animals)

Walking: Refer to page 86. Choose the ideal time of day for your schedule as well as where you will begin taking walks

☐ Morning before work

☐ Afternoon during lunch or break

☐ Evening before dinner or after

Writing: Refer to page 87. Find a special notebook or set up a private folder on your laptop so you can begin writing down your thoughts and feelings. Here are some questions below to get you started. For a writing worksheet, including a complete list of questions, refer to the bonus link.

• What 10 words best describe how I want to feel when I follow through with my *Heal Your Hunger* blueprint?

• What obstacles have stood in the way of my following through on proper self-care in the past (both inside and outside of myself)?

• How can I do things differently to ensure a more positive outcome?

Reading: Refer to page 90. Choose a few spiritual books you'd like to read from as part of your morning centeredness practice (*Refer also to the bonus Recommended Books & Readers.*)

Talking: Refer to page 91. Join the HYH community or identify a friend, relative, coach or therapist who has overcome emotional eating and with whom you can check in regularly.

☐ HYH community

☐ Friend

- ☐ Relative
- ☐ Coach
- ☐ Therapist

CLEAN EATING

Refer to page 95. Begin your 3 Meal Magic® plan by establishing regular times that you will eat each of your three meals and then check off the strategies you want to commit to in order to make 3 Meal Magic easier.

- ☐ Choose a time between 6am-9am _____
- ☐ Choose a time between 11pm-2pm _____
- ☐ Choose a time between 5pm-8pm _____
- ☐ **Prepare** your meals at home using fresh ingredients.
- ☐ **Eat** at the table.
- ☐ **Put** food on a plate—no eating from bags or boxes.
- ☐ **Don't** answer the phone while eating.
- ☐ **Refrain** from eating while driving.
- ☐ **Put** down your fork and breathe between bites.
- ☐ **Devote** 30-60 min for meals.
- ☐ **Write, talk and pray** about feelings that come up between meals.

COMMUNICATION

Refer to page 116. Practice speaking up by using the *10 Secrets to Expressing Yourself with Confidence*. Choose the 3 most important "secrets" and identify situations where you will practice each one. *(Refer to your 10 Secrets cheat sheet.)*

CONSCIOUSNESS-RAISING CONCEPTS

Refer to page 130. List which three concepts you will start to practice now and list them. *(You can also refer to your cheat sheet)*

CAUSES

Begin to examine the SOURCE when you are restless and feel "hungry". Check this list, put pen to paper and answer the questions below. See if you can begin to identify what's really going on:

Spiritual Void

☐ Am I disconnected from my spiritual source?

☐ Am I trying to do things on my own, without asking for help?

☐ Do I act and believe as if it all depends on me, forgetting that God is ready to help when I turn it over to him?

Old Wounds

☐ If I'm feeling hysterical, is this historical?

☐ If this is feeling like déjà vu, explore this by writing about when you have felt this way in the past.

☐ What situations from your childhood made you feel the same way?

☐ What happened and how did you feel as a kid when you went through that?

Untrue Beliefs

Are you operating under one of these beliefs or fears:

☐ I'm not smart enough.

☐ I'm never going to be successful.

☐ Things will always be tough.

☐ There isn't enough money.

- [ ] There isn't enough time.
- [ ] Someone will win and I'll lose.
- [ ] Someone will get mine.
- [ ] Good things never happen to me.
- [ ] I'm a bad person and deserve to be punished.
- [ ] Everybody hates me.
- [ ] I will die if I feel: fill in the blank…rejected, hungry, unloved, etc.

Resentment

- [ ] Whom do I resent and why?
- [ ] List all the ways you perceive they've hurt you.
- [ ] Did I play any part in the situation?
- [ ] Have I ever acted in the same way?
- [ ] Was it possible that that person acted from fear?
- [ ] Can I find it in my heart to forgive him or her?

Compromise

- [ ] Where in my life am I compromising myself, my values, my aspirations?
- [ ] Have I let go of certain goals on account of settling for less?
- [ ] Where in my life am I feeling dissatisfied and frustrated?

Ego

- [ ] Do I have a superior attitude toward anyone?
- [ ] Am I being self-righteous?
- [ ] Do I spend too much time on superficial things?
- [ ] Am I trying to control or change others?
- [ ] Am I attempting to force my will on a situation?

COURAGE

Refer to the list starting on page 158. Choose three courageous actions you will take as you begin your *Heal Your Hunger* path. *(For en**courage**ment, refer to the cheat sheet of famous quotes about courage.)*

★ ★ ★

Patience and persistence are the keys to success. There will be challenges, but what would life be without challenges that help us grow? If you fall, brush yourself off and get right back on the horse (or lion!) Take it one day at a time.

You don't have to do this alone. I'm here to support you.

The key is to embrace this healing path and the invaluable lessons it can teach you. Believe it or not, you can actually have fun with this. And you can experience freedom like nothing you've ever imagined.

It's time.

You've got this.

emotional
EATING
progression & recovery

(To be read left to right) © 2017 by Tricia Nelson

Progression

Emotional Eating

Food Addiction

- Low self esteem
- Big personality
- People-pleasing
- Overdoing
- Overspending
- Victim thinking
- Self-pity
- Depression
- Anxiety/panic attacks
- Resentment & blaming
- TV addiction
- Money problems
- Social phobias
- Hypertension
- Sleep apnea
- Isolation
- Insomnia
- Physical impairment
- Loss of job
- Prescription use

- Large appetite
- Constant nibbling
- Drawn to carbs, sugar and fat
- Obsession with food
- Loss of ordinary will power
- Binge-eating
- Nighttime eating
- Lying about food eaten
- Failed diets
- Vomiting/laxative abuse
- Extreme exercise
- Eating out of garbage
- Liposuction
- Geographical escapes
- Neglect of personal hygiene
- Diabetes
- Weight loss surgery

Can't stop destructive behaviors ⟶

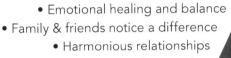

- Emotional healing and balance
- Family & friends notice a difference
- Harmonious relationships
- Frequent feelings of gratitude
- More comfortable in social situations
- Desire to be helpful to others
- Self-esteem grows
- Clear boundaries with others
- Confident self-expression
- Care of personal appearance
- Self-honesty
- Face fears
- Learn to say "no"
- Stop using food for emotional support

- Cravings are lifted
- Embrace reality (no longer escaping)
- Take responsibility for your life and healing
- Address underlying causes through SOURCE
- Integrate "6 Self-Care Success Secrets"
- 3 Meal Magic®
- Connect regularly with those on the HYH path
- Re-prioritize your schedule
- Feeling of safety and belonging
- Join the HYH community
- Learn that it's an inside job
- Sincere desire to get help

Heal Your Hunger

← ——— **Seeking help**

ACKNOWLEDGMENTS

I am eternally grateful to the many people who helped make this book a reality.

To Roy Nelson, my husband, mentor, and teacher, and the living embodiment of the principles in this book, all of which you taught me and helped me implement in my own life. God knew what he was doing that day in November 1987, when I was blessed to hear you speak and you touched my heart.

To my intelligent, funny, loving, heart-centered friends who helped me edit this book and provided invaluable feedback and endless moral support: Tsilah Burman, Kim Hamer, Antoinette Bryant, Elizabeth Kelley Erickson, Linda Victor, Dawnmarie Fitzgerald, and Tanna Frederick.

To my late father, Ed Greaves, who inspires me every day to do my best and to give to this world as he did every day of his life. I love you, Daddy.

To my Mom, Connie Greaves Bates, who is a true gift in my life. Thank you for your joie de vivre, for your unconditional love, and for proving that thinking of others is the best antiaging secret there is. I love you.

To my sisters, Jenn and Carolyn, for always loving me and cheering me on.

To all my friends, family, and teachers, thank you for helping me realize more and more each day how connected we all are and how good God is.

To Michael Fishman and Elaine Glass, thank you for your vision of what must be.

To my amazing book muse, Lisa Canfield, my brilliant editor, Michael Carr, my awesome graphic designers, Adele Wiejaczka and Jodi Voegele, and my talented cartoonist, Mariano Pogoriles. Thank you for making this book shine.

To Mary Agnes Antonopoulos and Team, thank you for your heart and hard work in helping me reach those who most need this message.

To all the clients who have been a part of our lives over the past three decades. Thank you for illuminating what it really means to be an emotional eater and for proving the efficacy of these seven simple steps.

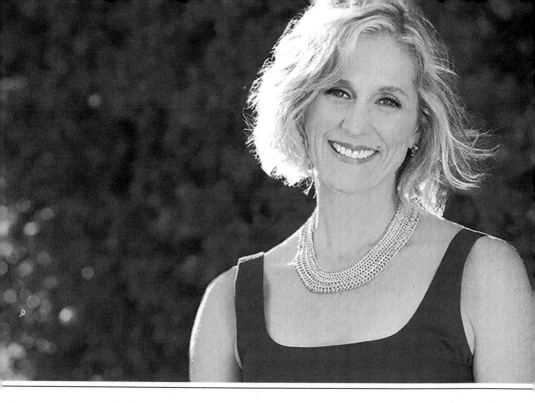

Tricia Nelson grew up in Concord, Massachusetts, and received her degree from Amherst College. In her early 20s Tricia lost fifty pounds and transformed her life by identifying and healing the underlying causes of her emotional eating. She has spent nearly thirty years researching the hidden causes of the addictive personality. Together with her husband, spiritual healer Roy Nelson, she has helped hundreds of people overcome their food addiction and other addictions. Tricia is an Emotional Eating Expert and host of the popular podcast **The Heal Your Hunger Show**. A highly regarded speaker and coach, Tricia has been featured on NBC, CBS, KTLA, FOX, and Discovery Health. She resides in Los Angeles with her husband.

**To access this book's bonus material and companion course
go to www.healyourhungerbook.com**

---

www.HealYourHunger.com

✻

800.609.4061

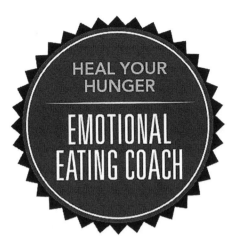

HEAL YOUR HUNGER ADVANCED TRAINING FOR HEALTH COACHES AND PRACTITIONERS

I want to help every person who struggles with food and weight to finally experience freedom from emotional eating, but I cannot do this alone.

For this reason, I have created a training that will empower health coaches and practitioners with the tools, education and step-by-step system they can use to guide their clients to freedom. This is the exact system I have used to help thousands of clients around the world.

To learn more about my professional-level program and how you can use the Heal Your Hunger method to support your clients and community, as well as increase revenue and impact, please access my FREE TRAINING.

**To access this FREE TRAINING, please go to
www. HYHCoachTraining.com**

Made in the USA
San Bernardino, CA
22 August 2018